D1826140

CHOOSE HEALTH—CHOOSE LIFE

Kenneth Vickery qualified in 1941 proceeding to the most senior medical degree of his university (MD London) in 1947. He was House Physician at St Bartholomew's Hospital London (1941–42) and Medical Officer RAMC (1942–46) attaining the rank of Major with responsibilities in Army Health and Hygiene in Jerusalem.

Following further post-war qualifications in Public Health he was appointed Deputy Medical Officer of Health, Bournemouth, and subsequently Medical Officer of Health for the County Borough of Eastbourne. He served as a Member of the Council of the Soil Association in the fifties, and on the Council of the Royal Society of Health during the seventies. He was Chairman of the Council of the Royal Institute of Public Health from 1976 to 1982 and received the Smith Award of that Royal Institute for service to the public health.

Dr Vickery is currently Honorary Consultant in Public Health and Vice-President of the Royal Institute of Public Health and an Officer of the Order of St John of Jerusalem.

He has over some forty years written and spoken extensively to the health professions and the public of his conviction that nutritional deficiency is the major underlying cause of so much of the ill-health which besets Western society. He has also consistently advocated public policies to sustain the integrity of the living soil as the source of fresh food so essential to the public health.

Choose Health – Choose Life

KENNETH VICKERY
OStJ, MD, FFCM, DPH

Foreword by Ian Gow TD, MP

KINGSWAY PUBLICATIONS
EASTBOURNE

Copyright © Kenneth Vickery 1986

First published 1986

All rights reserved.
No part of this publication may be reproduced or
transmitted in any form or by any means, electronic
or mechanical, including photocopy, recording, or any
information storage and retrieval system, without
permission in writing from the publisher.

ISBN 0 86065 388 9

Unless otherwise indicated, biblical quotations are from
the Authorized Version, crown copyright

RSV = Revised Standard Version
copyrighted 1946, 1952, © 1971, 1973 by the
Division of Christian Education of the National
Council of the Churches of Christ in the USA

NIV = New International Version
© New York International Bible Society 1978

Front cover photo: Tony Stone Photolibrary

Printed in Great Britain for
KINGSWAY PUBLICATIONS LTD
Lottbridge Drove, Eastbourne, E. Sussex BN23 6NT by
Richard Clay Ltd, Bungay, Suffolk.
Typeset by CST, Eastbourne, E. Sussex.

Contents

Conservation of soil, water, waste and trees—
Political objectives

Acknowledgements

My chapters 'Apostles of Health' and 'Journey into Health and Life' form part of an expression of great indebtedness. My appreciation is also further due for specific encouragement and personal communications relating to this task to Dr Denis Burkitt FRS, Surg., Commander Brian Cliff OBE and to Mrs Doris Grant. Also here in Eastbourne to Dr Vincent Harris for so kindly reading the script and providing invaluable advice in matters medical, spiritual and literary.

My thanks also to Mr K. R. Ryan, administrative officer and librarian, Royal Naval Hospital, Plymouth, for most helpful information and advice in the pursuit of historical detail. Also to Mr David Trigger, Curator of the Museum, Royal William Victualling Yard, Plymouth in regard to nineteenth-century diet and custom in the Royal Navy. Also to Mr Andrew Baster of the Wills Library, Guys Hospital, London for historical information.

In the onerous tasks of type, word and print my most grateful thanks are due to Eileen Boniface for typescript and literary advice and to my wife Nancy for the same. Also to Jacqui Dann for typing and clerical help.

Foreword

Dr Kenneth Vickery's achievements and teaching in the field of health are well-known within and around my constituency. Those achievements and that teaching are known too, to doctors in the Public Health Service. With their support, he has held office nationally, and is the holder of a Public Health 'Oscar'.

I am honoured to have the opportunity of commending this book to a wider audience. I do so with confidence, because of Dr Vickery's long experience. He has been ahead of his time in perceiving and in advancing the priorities which really matter in the promotion of health. He considers healthy eating to be the most important of all. For some forty years he has been calling for changes which, until very lately, were received only hesitatingly by the health professions. He was arguing for adequate roughage in our food long before the recent 'discovery' of bran.

Dr Vickery came to Eastbourne as Medical Officer of Health some thirty-five years ago. Shortly after his arrival he set up one of the first centres in the UK for health education of the public. Priority was given to expectant and nursing mothers and to children. His teaching, shared with an enthusiastic staff, encouraged the value of whole, fresh food and the avoidance of excess sugar and refined food. At that time such teaching was unique.

In the early sixties the first comprehensive health centre of any health resort in Britain was established, facilitating close co-operation of the health team with the family doctors. Later one of the first community dietitians was appointed. With the support of the former County Borough Council, Dr Vickery also developed some of the most effective caring services in Britain for the elderly and for the handicapped, including their special needs for nourishing food.

By a strange incidence of events, I am able to vouch for an even earlier chapter of the author's pedigree. In the early years of World War 2, Kenneth Vickery was completing his medical training at one of our most famous teaching hospitals —St Bartholomew's or, as I have always known it, 'Barts'. He was appointed there as House Physician to my father who was then the Senior Consultant in Medicine.

Dr Vickery insists that I should not identify myself with all or any of his views or prescriptions. As a lawyer and politician it is probably inappropriate that I should do so. However, I am delighted that he has surrendered to the encouragement of his friends, colleagues and particularly of his family, to set down a way, as he sees it, to better health. That way is standing the test of time and will be developed much further in the years that lie ahead. I am also very pleased that publication is being undertaken by Kingsway, the international publishers whose activities are such a considerable asset to my constituency.

Dr Vickery explains that preventive medicine and the promotion of health are worthy pursuits. In the Book of Ecclesiasticus we are advised: 'Honour a physician with the honour due unto him, for the uses which ye may have of him: for the Lord hath created him.' Our familiar use of the physician is when we fall sick, where his ministrations can be a godsend. It is all too easy for us to overlook an even more important use—that of helping us to avoid falling ill. This is his role as teacher, which is the very meaning of the title 'doctor', and reminds us of that greatest of teachers, Luke, described by St Paul in his letter to the Colossians as 'the beloved physician'.

All of which lends point to the wise advice in the Book of

Ecclesiasticus (New English Bible translation): 'Before you fall sick consult a doctor.' This encourages me to share the author's purpose in seeking to secure better health as part of that more abundant life promised by Christ himself.

IAN GOW, TD, MP
House of Commons

*I have set before you life and death . . .
therefore choose life.*
                    (Deuteronomy 30:19)

*Life is only known as the complex of
many functions, and health as the integrity of these functions, each in itself,
and their harmony among the others.*
                    PETER M. LATHAM (1789-1875)

INTRODUCTION

Healthwise through the Jungle

'Oh Shut Up All You Experts!'
'Eat Your Words You Doctors!'
'Down With Killjoys!'
'Eyewash!' (Everything You Enjoy Will Affect Sound Health.)
'Fed Up With Food Fads!'
'Polyunsaturated Poppycock!'
'So Healthy—So Boring!'
'We Want Prescriptions, Not Patter!'

These are cries from the heart and are but a few from my collection of outbursts of public exasperation as the health lobbies vie with each other and with the food industry. They are captions from readers' letters in the national press. They predictably appear whenever the pundits come out with the latest cautionary health advice, especially when it is centred upon some time-honoured foodstuff. Invariably a centenarian will also be quoted as having broken this and every other rule of health for a lifetime.

The newspaper columnists and headline writers thrive on these controversies. A not unusual line is that there is a Puritan conspiracy to deprive us of what we enjoy, or to make us feel guilty. A typical opinion is that it is more important that people should be free to eat junk than that they should be bossed to eat well (Mary Kenny, *Daily Mail*, October 9th 1985).

Collectively these public and press reactions should be the ultimate deterrent for all official and self-appointed experts— particularly doctors like me—from making a statement, appearing on TV or writing a book—especially writing a book!

Why do it then? There have surely been more than enough books and television programmes. Yes, but unfortunately they are nearly all about disease, its fascination and its treatment, with large helpings of the workings of the inner recesses of the body (courtesy of fibre optics). We are beset with disease but there has been far too little understanding of health; how to achieve it and how to stay with it.

The seeker of health is beset by a jungle of conflicting and mostly disease-orientated advice. In the pages that follow we will be searching out the common denominators of health, where they are to be found in nature, and to establish basic principles of healthy ways of living. It is my hope that you will then be encouraged to see that the attainment of health is very much in our own hands, and that, having recognized what rings true, you will feel able to act upon it. Of course we need to keep a balanced perspective on life as a whole and pursue healthy living without obsession, hypochondria or undue anxiety.

I intend to show that the greater part of the appalling burden of disease which afflicts civilized man, in contrast to the relative health of wildlife, is a direct consequence of damaging habits of living. We will see that, by simple changes, health can be improved and future liability to disease diminished. The changes will be mainly concerned with our daily eating habits and will not involve unacceptably restrictive diets. New types of food will, after a period of adjustment, be found to be truly enjoyable. (From here on the use of the word 'diet' will denote a variety of foods we choose, rather than a regime imposed upon us.)

A starvation of quality will be shown to be at the heart of our food deficiencies. At the same time we will not overlook the fact that for major parts of the Third World there is little choice of quality or quantity.

The briefest definition of health is the one most suited to be our watchword along the way: 'wholeness'. I shall be pleading that one of the greatest handicaps to man's progress, out of the baleful morass of disease in which he struggles, is an incredible built-in propensity to tunnel vision. Man is never happier than when creating multiple specialities. His experts are disinclined to look sideways, finding the language of other specialities increasingly perplexing. The key to the understanding of health will be shown to be ecology. That is a consideration of man's health in relation to the health of the living species about him and the total environment. A word, if only for the purposes of reproach, is required to describe the blinkered vision which is the precise opposite of this concept. The meaning of an old English word might fittingly be extended for this purpose: 'monology'.

If I claim to have been driven to bringing these observations of a lifetime together by anguish, I risk losing credibility. But I cannot deny that I have been utterly saddened and sickened by the perpetuation of massive and tragic disease while the knowledge necessary for prevention has been available and progressively enlarged for at least a hundred years—indeed for thousands of years in the case of some diseases, as we shall see. For those for whom it may be helpful to know a little more of what has led me to this exposition, I have preferred to undertake this towards the end of the book in chapter 15.

Adding life to the years

We must be mindful that the invitation 'choose health', although intended to be an encouragement for the majority, might seem to be callous for a minority already severely handicapped or suffering from grave chronic or degenerative disease. For such, and for many in the hinterland between disease and health, I will maintain that at whatever point we start, and at whatever age, there is a potential for preventing the worsening of established disease, the possibility of improvement and, at the very least, if not adding years to life, of adding life to the years remaining.

The years remaining: this is the crunch of the matter. In this physical and temporal existence these will, at best, amount to the tiniest fragment of the aeons of time of the universe. Can that really be all there is in it for us, whether in good health or bad?

Health we shall see comprises not only the physical but also the mental and spiritual. This is a concept instinctively felt by many, and widely and long endorsed by doctors and clergy. I will be looking at that spiritual dimension in a Christian context. I do not apologize for this, and I hope that those readers who do not share my spiritual outlook will nonetheless be encouraged to see that there is more to life than physical existence, and that when Jesus Christ promised his followers 'abundant life' he was referring to a quality of life which transcends our earthly existence.

For this reason the scope and title of the book does not stop at the invitation 'choose health', but continues on in the latter chapters to encouragement of the much more tremendous and enduring opportunity to 'choose life'.

When meditating over a disease I never think of finding a remedy, but instead a means of prevention.

LOUIS PASTEUR (1884)

I

Grievous Bodily Harm

We recoil in horror when we read about sudden grievous bodily harm, mugging, wife beating and baby battering. Yet millions of us are party to grievous harm to our own bodies and those we care for, by faulty habits of living—most of all through choosing or providing the wrong food.

An anxious mother and her three eldest children made their way into the ward of the grey stone building of the Royal Naval Hospital, Plymouth. Her husband and their father lay ashen faced, knees drawn up and a vomit bowl by his side. From his movements, he was evidently in considerable internal pain, in spite of the laudanum which was being liberally administered.

This was the last time they were to see their dear one alive. Following a long voyage from the East, involving considerable deprivations during and after the Egypt/Sudan campaign, Albert had been rowed from his ship in a pinnace along the Stonehouse Creek to the hospital quay. Little more could, in fact, be done for him in hospital than at sea. He was almost certainly suffering from acute perforated appendicitis. His abdomen was tender and full of pus. He required surgical intervention and drainage. But the year was 1887 and only a very few brave attempts at surgery for this condition had yet been undertaken worldwide. Indeed, the very term 'appendicitis' had not been adopted until the previous year. One of the earliest successful operations was in 1902 upon King Edward

VII, whose coronation was postponed because of his condition.

We know that on long voyages the food of mariners at that time was very restricted: salted meat, hard tack, bread and puddings made with refined flour, together with a liberal use of sugar and treacle. There was little, if any, vegetable or fruit. Wholemeal flour would not keep at sea, being subject to mould and weevils. Dietary fibre, essential for healthy working of the bowel, was singularly lacking. Acute appendicitis was certainly one disease which flourished on this deprived fodder. Kidney disease—under the general description of Bright's disease—was also prevalent, arising from prolonged and excessive exposure to salted food.

Albert had gone to sea as a robust son of Devon. He had survived earlier shipwreck in cold seas, having swum many miles to the shore, but slowly and surely his health was undermined. It was cut short that night, at the age of thirty-seven, leaving a widow and five children. He was a victim of his time and of what I now choose to call Deplete Food Disease. He was also my grandfather.

The stress of his tragic early demise upon the family was such that the events were well remembered and handed down —such as his funeral service in the newly-built Church of the Good Shepherd in the Royal Naval Hospital, and the procession with muffled drums to the RN burial ground at No Place Field nearby. Among the details retold by an elderly relative while I was a medical student was the stated cause of death— 'Bright's disease and Typhlitis'. I had to look in a very old textbook to find the latter which I now realize was a term used for inflammation of the bowel before the nature of appendicitis was properly understood.

I quote his case to illustrate that Deplete Food Disease (which I will define later) was already established 100 years ago, and was something to which mariners were especially prone.

If thy bowel offend thee, cut it out

We move forward almost a quarter of a century to 1910. Gow-land Hopkins was not to discover the B Vitamins until 1912. None but a few 'cranks' prized the brown germ and bran of wheat and rice. Sugar was cheap and abundant. Fruit and vegetables were not universally popular, had a very limited season, and were little valued in terms of health.

Deplete Food Disease was rampant. Its precursor, consti-pation or costiveness, as it was called, was widespread and at times very disabling. Like the case of the bishop's wife. Her symptoms were so bad she found herself in the Harley Street rooms of a distinguished London surgeon, having been refer-red there by her country doctor. 'It's been a burden for most of my life, doctor,' she admitted with evident embarrassment. 'Dreadful when I was carrying the children and now, as the years go by, worse and worse. Life seems to be a constant round of senna, cascara, croton oil and the enema.'

On examination, the surgeon felt a hard elongated mass in the abdomen and a complete stoppage of solid excrement in the back passage. 'I expect your doctor told you that if I were to help it would mean surgery?'

'Well, yes,' she replied, 'he told me you had perfected a relief operation.'

'I expect he also told you the risks?' The risk of death was, in fact, at least one in five!

The surgeon was William Arbuthnot Lane, who gave his name to an operation involving complete removal of the greater part of the large bowel, short circuiting the small bowel to the back passage—a procedure to become known as 'Lane's Loop'. Lane was later to be elevated to Sir William, following a successful operation upon a princess.

The bishop's wife survived the operation. Her immediate symptoms were alleviated but were exchanged for tiresome unpredictable bowel habits; she became very anaemic and never felt really well again. Today she would be told that a sufficiency of food roughage is essential for healthy bowel action, but the poor lady received no such advice then, nor have millions before or since.

To his eternal credit, by 1925 Sir William Arbuthnot Lane, Bart., had seen the light. He had concluded that many of the conditions upon which he had operated were fundamentally preventable. He laid down his scalpel to embark upon health education of the public. His battle against professional prejudice, and the price he paid, merits further mention in chapter 12.

Pregnancy—nature's diet efficiency test

Taking a further leap of twenty-five years from 1910, ignorance concerning food and health continued to abound in 1935. Millions caught up in the poverty of the depression subsisted on appalling food: white bread, cakes, pastry, puddings, biscuits made from deprived white flour. Sugar, in its many forms, was being consumed in excess of 100lbs per person per year. Adequate vegetables and fruit were beyond the means of many. Those who could afford better were inhibited by ignorance.

There were a few voices, a very few, crying in the wilderness. Like the group of doctors in Cheshire who in 1939 issued a 'Medical Testament' deploring the state of the nation's health and linking it squarely with poor food. 'Our daily work,' they exclaimed,

> brings us repeatedly to the same point—this illness results from a lifetime of wrong nutrition. The wrong nutrition begins before life begins: most of the ills we are called upon to attend are the result not only of wrong nutrition but also of inferior food, namely food grown on exhausted land—refined foods, deprived foods. Our further indictment is constipation—its cause is the choice or ill preparation of food. The prevention of sickness depends on right feeding.

Such was the climate when we meet our third patient in 1935. Two patients in fact, a mother and her baby.

Grace was the daughter of retired missionaries. She was

twenty-six and lived in an industrial town in the north of England. She had two children aged six and four. Although there was much poverty and unemployment in the district her husband had a secure job as a teacher in a church primary school. There was not much left for luxuries on his salary but they never went short of food—in terms of quantity at any rate.

Grace had had several miscarriages and two difficult pregnancies culminating in long, exhausting deliveries. She was now pregnant again and having a very bad time. She had gained weight rapidly and her ankles and other tissues were very swollen. She could no longer remove the ring on her finger. She was pale, listless and her morning sickness was the worst ever. As her time advanced she began to have fits of a kind similar to epilepsy. Her condition caused so much anxiety that she was admitted to a maternity hospital and labour was induced ahead of time. A sickly child was delivered, a boy, and was found to be suffering from spina bifida—a condition of incomplete development where the bony spinal column fails to unite at the back leaving the spinal nerves exposed. The child died after forty-eight hours; his mother was also dead within the week.

Records show that this type of tragedy was typical of thousands in the inter-war years. We know about Grace's case because of a particularly painstaking investigation by a young doctor from the department of the Medical Officer of Health where these deaths were notified. He had the co-operation of the sorrowing husband and Grace's mother who was now struggling with the two orphaned children.

The doctor was the son of a very enlightened general practitioner. The essence of his finding was that the mother had been suffering from toxaemia of pregnancy and anaemia, culminating in eclampsia, which is characterized by fits. He found that the food of the family was centred around bread, cakes, biscuits, puddings and cornflakes—all made from white flour and all liberally laced with jams and sugary confections. Fresh fruit and vegetables were singularly lacking as were the more expensive and body-building protein foods like meat, fish, eggs and cheese.

The young doctor noticed that her Christian parents, who had taught in undeveloped countries, had no basic knowledge of what constituted a healthy diet. Grace had had little or no instruction in school. Her antenatel care had not included any health education advice. He made little comment on the deformed baby, apart from the generalization that the young embryo had doubtless been lacking a sufficiency of nutrients at critical times during development.

It is now accepted, but only in very recent years, that the kind of developmental deformity of Grace's baby may be associated with a deficiency of a Vitamin of the B group known as folic acid. Mothers who have had a baby with spina bifida are increasingly being given vitamin supplements with subsequent pregnancies. This is typical of the piecemeal approach in the prevention of disease. Far better to advocate a wholefood fresh food diet for all expectant mothers. We certainly now know that the dietary fibre, despised and rejected in the thirties and until quite recent times, is of considerable importance in the prevention of toxaemia of pregnancy. Now, as was the case in the thirties, pregnancy is a 'diet efficiency' test. A diet which may not have caused serious problems in a nonpregnant adult may quickly prove insufficient in pregnancy. Raised blood pressure, swelling of the tissues, excessive weight gain can be tell-tale signs. Important as sound feeding is for any of us, it is imperative during pregnancy and breastfeeding, when great demands by the offspring are placed on the mother's stores of calcium, iron and other vital substances.

Sadly, Grace and her baby died from preventable conditions. They were victims of Deplete Food Disease.

The vicarage family

Health or disease is a matter which so often affects every member of the family—not merely the individual. Our fourth case history, twenty-five years later in 1960, reveals an entire family in poor health.

It was Sunday and we were on holiday in Cornwall. It was a glorious shining sunlit day as we made our way to the picturesque stone-built church within sight of the sea. The landscape was ablaze with early flowers. Lambs were flourishing in the rich pasture—truly a day which the Lord had given in which to rejoice. Surely health must abound in such luxuriant surroundings!

Yet, inside the lovely church, what struck us most forcibly was how ill the vicar looked. His face was drawn as he ascended into the pulpit; he appeared to be in pain from time to time. Further, deciding that the mother, three children and granny who came in by a side door constituted the rest of the vicarage family, we could not help but remark how ill they also looked.

Much as we often long to get alongside a sickly family, we have learned not to proffer advice unless it is asked for, and then only in terms of health education unlikely to offend any possible doctor/patient relationship.

As things turned out a midweek event in the church hall renewed contact with the vicar. 'Saw you on Sunday,' he said. 'Where are you from?' 'Eastbourne,' I replied, and this elicited, as it so often does, a mutual acquaintance, and the fact that we were in the health business soon emerged. One thing led to another and we were graciously invited to high tea at the vicarage later in the week.

We were right about the ill health. They seemed anxious to talk. Father's health was giving the most immediate concern. A long history now of abdominal pain, flatulence, heartburn and distension, repeated investigations and the ever-present threat of surgery.

'Di . . . something they think.'

'Diverticular disease,' we mused.

'Yes, that's it. That's what the x-rays confirmed. They say it's getting very common these days.'

All three children had suffered a particularly bad winter

and considerable absence from school due to repeated coughs and colds, sore throats, discharging ears, dental abcess and a fractured arm from a most trivial fall. Mother admitted also that she never really felt well. She attributed some of it to being overweight—something she felt unable to control. Constipation was a common denominator of the whole family. Granny was also overweight and suffered painful joints.

They had provided a generous tea for us and it would seem ungracious to comment adversely. However, if this was typical of the household food habits, we realized that we would have to grasp the nettle! Much of the food was evidently home baked but every item—sandwiches, sausage rolls, scones, and sponge cake—was prepared with white bread or white flour. There was considerable added sugar in the form of jam, icing, orange drinks and sweetened tea.

Here again was Deplete Food Disease.

We were privileged to keep in touch with the family and to help along the lines of chapter 6. There was a progressive improvement in their health. Much to his doctor's surprise, Father's abdominal discomfiture went away without an operation, which was as well since results of orthodox treatment, including surgery, were at that time very unsatisfactory.

Diverticular disease of the large bowel is a twentieth-century scourge. Society is considerably indebted to Mr Neil Painter MS, FRCS, who devised and pursued surgical experimentation which at last gives hope of alleviation and prevention. Against the trend of orthodox opinion he has related this condition, whose precursor is constipation, to a deprivation of adequate roughage in the food. Yet another manifestation of Deplete Food Disease.

The whole family now join Father in taking simple miller's bran. They bake their own wholemeal bread. They make yoghurt from the abundant local milk. They grow more fruit and vegetables.

The children are more resistant to infection and winter ailments. Mother recognizes that the health of the family is more in her hands than she ever realized. Granny swears by the bran and has also lost weight. Her mobility is improved, although her arthritis is too far gone to be significantly reversed.

Indifferent food was a far more weighty factor in the health of this family than the sea air, sun, lovely climate and their comfortable home. A family can be healthy in a hovel or, with the wrong food, unhealthy in a palace—or a vicarage with roses round the door.

By 1960 there were still at least twenty years to elapse before there was to be any real awakening in the health professions towards a more healthy diet. Indeed, a leading article that year in *The Lancet,* one of the top journals for doctors, stated:

> There are hardly any signs yet that doctors and dentists care enough about nutrition to set their weight firmly against the commercial interests concerned . . . the day may be far distant when the public can be weaned from its present somewhat infantile over-dependence on refined sugar.

Our final leap of twenty-five years brings us to 1985 to consider the case of Alice. She was a very active housewife of sixty-five, until one day she stood on a stair that wasn't there and fractured the long bone of the hip joint at its weakest point.

The fall which caused the break seemed relatively trivial. It is of course well known that with advancing years, and for females in particular, some loss of the substance of the bones takes place. This is partly associated with glandular changes. I am bound to say, however (and this view is shared by an eminent orthopaedic surgeon of my acquaintance), that a factor in this fragility of the bones is due to a shortage of organically-bound minerals in the food. When we consider the tea and biscuits diet of many old people, this is not hard to believe. Certainly, on enquiry, Alice's food was not very 'enlightened'—although rather better than many of the thousands of elderly ladies living alone. But then she had a husband to feed!

Indeed the same orthopaedic surgeon, commenting upon

the late twentieth-century epidemic of backache and sciatica, points to the shock-absorber pads between the spinal bones. He finds they have decayed like the teeth and, instead of the expected hard resiliant substance, have collapsed, causing the nerves to be compressed and to protest. His view of the fundamental cause of the decay of these intervertebral discs and other bones would justify their inclusion in our concept of Deplete Food Disease.

However, orthopaedic surgeons are very skilled at fixing bones around the hip joint and Alice seemed to make an immediate recovery. Nevertheless an early consequence of the operation was a complete loss of bowel activity. On the fifth day, in spite of the efforts of the physiotherapist, there were signs of blood clotting in the leg and pelvis. She died suddenly on the seventh day from pulmonary embolism. A clot of blood detached from the veins below had blocked a major artery supplying the lungs. She joined about 4,000 others who die prematurely each year in the UK from this cause.

There is a well-demonstrated over-filling and stagnation of the large bowel whenever people are confined to bed. Motions passed tend to be at best an overflow. The loaded bowel presses upon the big veins receiving blood from the lower limbs. Clotting occurs all too easily. Some surgeons and ward sisters, at long last, arrange for patients coming in for an operation to take simple miller's bran for a few days previously. This bran is continued into convalescence.

Alice died prematurely in 1985 as a result of Deplete Food Disease—just as surely as my grandfather did in 1887. The disease was incriminated in each of these sample cases, typical of millions who also suffered grievous bodily harm during that span of 100 years, and who sadly continue to succumb. Will we never learn?

Postscript

On the very day I completed this chapter I received papers

relating to a lady who died in hospital from a painful, distressing but perfectly preventable condition. Her death certificate reads: 'Acute peritonitis, due to perforation of the large bowel, due to chronic constipation.'

Nurture determines the extent to which we can achieve the upper limits of well-being set by Nature. While no one would want to underestimate the influence of modern medicine, good housing and other environmental conditions, in promoting good health, everyone can be sure that food comes first.

HAZEL K. STIEBELING
U.S. Dept of Agriculture Yearbook (1959)

2

Deplete Food Disease

Deplete Food Disease, which is the unrelenting consequence of faulty food habits, has continued to exact an appalling toll of disease and premature death right up to the present day. It was not until 1983 that there began to be any significant professional response to the long-held contention of a minority that all is very far from well with our national food habits. But there was not yet any agreed health education programme, even to start to put things right—in sharp contrast with the USA which had been propagating the agreed McGovern Dietary Goals for the US for at least eight years.

In January 1985 *The Observer* of Great Britain fired a timely broadside at the continuing inertia—public, professional and commercial—and again underlined the shortcomings and sophistication of so much of our food and the poor choice we make overall. The contentions were made that no more than a third of what we eat is good for us and, as a nation, we are now as badly fed as we were fifty years ago.

Manning *The Observer's* guns were Geoffrey Cannon and Caroline Walker, whose book *The Food Scandal* had recently been published. History may well confirm that their contribution was crucial in the battle for the British diet and that 1985 was the turning point. Certainly there were continuing reverberations in the media throughout the year, including major TV and radio documentaries.

Cannon and Walker's carefully researched facts, and the

sense of urgency in their expression, deserved immediate encouragement. I am sure they received it from many quarters, but it happened that my letter under the heading 'Healthy food for thought' was the support which was published in *The Observer*. In this I also specified the long-felt need for public awareness of deprivation of food at all points in the food chain and for a descriptive term embracing the numerous and serious manifestations of common cause arising from Western food deficiency. The term I proposed was 'Deplete Food Disease'.

The twilight state

I now refer also to a less advanced state of ill-health which I describe as 'Deplete Food Profile'. This I see as a state of impending ill-health in which, during latent or incubation periods, a large part of the peoples of the West are unwittingly existing. I am confirmed in this assessment by the observations of that great reforming nutritionist, Dr Max O. Bircher-Benner, who more than half a century ago described a state of 'twilight zone of ill-health'.

Circumstantial evidence

I felt justified and entitled to support *The Observer's* description of our food deficiencies, and to put a name to the consequences, having contended as much publicly for some forty years. Specifically, in a paper presented to a public conference in Bournemouth, in 1953, I pointed to impoverished sophisticated food as the biggest single cause of disease in the West. I drew attention to mounting deficiencies of vital and trace substances and specified that the health professionals must become ecologists if any real progress was to be made in the promotion of health.

I had arrived at these conclusions in no small part as a result of the travel and observations mentioned in chapter 15; also taking into account the unexpected post-Second World War findings that, in spite of grave shortages of food in European countries, certain serious diseases had been less prevalent. Subsequently work in the Public Health Service enabled me to undertake medical examinations upon some thousands of school children, toddlers, infants and babies. I was able to question them and their parents about their living habits and daily food. The opportunity was taken, whenever possible, to visit them at home and assess the food in the larder. I was looking primarily for signs of health in the children, but was appalled at the prevalence of bad teeth and mouth structure, poor facial and dental arch form, septic tonsils, running ears, spinal curvature, winged shoulder blades, septic skin conditions, constipation—and the inevitable school absenteeism resulting from all this ill health.

I was also influenced by the apparently ignored results of some thousands of scientific papers—published worldwide—incriminating one or more vital substance or trace element with significant occurrence of disease. In paper after paper the authors sought to show that if this, that or the other missing nutrient was restored to the diet as a treatment, recovery would ensue. A classic example in 1952 was the discovery, in Australia, that shortage of fibre in the diet predisposed one to the selfsame diseases of pregnancy suffered by Grace (chapter 1). But no one took any notice!

Indeed, no one seemed to be making any attempt to link these suspected deficiency diseases together and to wonder if the diet was not deficient overall. Intriguingly, over the same period, horticulturalists, farmers and veterinary surgeons were making very similar observations arising from deficiency in plants, crops and animals. Commercial concern prompted much more rapid progress than was the case with human health.

Professional inhibition

Why, it must be asked, did we have to go on tolerating food deficiency and consequent disease for so many long years and do next to nothing about it?

The first reason is man's overall resistance to any change in the established way of doing things, typified by the ingrained food habits handed down from mother to daughter. Second is the established practice of food producers and manufacturers detailed in the next chapter.

The third great hindrance—and I record it with sorrow—is the position and attitude of the medical profession. All doctors start with the handicap that their whole training is orientated to the study, detection and treatment of disease. The clamouring demands of disease occupy the greater part of the working life of most doctors. Only a very small number are engaged in preventive medicine or have the opportunity to look at health and to consider the common ingredients of healthy individuals, healthy families and healthy communities.

White mouse medicine

The further handicap of the medical profession is a slavish adherence to what has been described and deplored by that great British physician and surgeon, Sir Heneage Ogilvie, as 'white mouse medicine'. This largely arises from immersion in disease. Cranks, quacks and charlatans have flourished down the years with new and untried treatments for gullible patients. It has become a discipline that no change in established practice for any treatment shall be recognized unless and until there have been repeated controlled experiments. These often commence with laboratory animals before being tentatively tried out on patients. There are usually built-in safeguards to rule out extraneous factors and we hear the term 'double-blind trials' (see glossary).

These same requirements have been held to be necessary before the medical profession is able to lend its support to any change in diet or food habit for the individual, or the public at large. Unfortunately, however, controlled trials simply do not lend themselves to the drawing of deductions upon what is, or is not, a healthy diet. Such trials are almost impossible to devise, because it is so notoriously difficult to control the many variables in human behaviour. There have been very few positive results, with the consequence that a majority of doctors have felt inhibited to proffer advice on healthy eating to the well or the sick.

Another inexcusable delay

Indeed it was not until the results of one of the most extensive controlled trials ever that the body of the profession came to recognize that habits of living might have a significant effect upon health. I refer to the work which was eventually able to validate the obvious conclusion that smoking was bad for health. I say 'obvious' because hundreds of doctors observing thousands of patients over many years had already reached the conclusion that there is a direct association between smoking and lung disease, including cancer of the lung. But they were never able to express a collective view on the matter and, if they had, it would have been challenged as unscientific.

So an addicted public and the flower of its youth had to wait for decades—until at least 1962—pending evidence, served up in the statistical manner beloved of the scientific journals, before anyone dare say something to the effect that 'a majority of doctors consider that smoking is harmful to health'. Earlier action could have saved thousands of lives and much disease. It is fortunate, however, that this marathon of research on smoking and health was carried out—and even pursued to the extent of proving that smoking fifty to sixty cigarettes a day was more damaging than thirty to forty. The professional mind was at last open to the possibility that other living habits, such as diet, might affect health. Even so, in regard to smoking, notwithstanding some of the most painstaking, prolonged and exhaustive research ever conducted, numerous red herrings are drawn across the trail by doctors and others who will not be convinced. If decisive research such as this can be doubted, we can see what we are up against in getting food habits changed!

So it is that uncorrected bad habits have continued throughout the twentieth century to engender grievous bodily disease. It has not been possible to contrive controlled experiments to 'prove' the day-to-day observations of numerous intelligent persons, professional and lay.

We have been too slow to pool the consensus of observations and to accept the tool of epidemiology in the study of families and races in health and disease. Meanwhile, in a climate of disease which shows no abatement, we continue to 'fiddle while Rome burns' instead of modifying our lifestyles to profit from the examples of good health which have been found in the laboratory of nature.

Crass observational blindness

The story of dietary fibre provides one of the saddest and most damaging examples of inertia and prejudice. From the time when roughage first began to be significantly lost from man's food, there have been keen observers who could see the baleful consequences upon health—some of which were quite obvious. The beginning of that time was at least 150 years ago, when white flour and white bread had become the order of the day for the majority. The consequences of the fibre loss were further aggravated, about fifty years later, by the rapidly rising consumption of another carbohydrate food from which all the fibre had been extracted: sugar.

Time and time again over the years a few perceptive voices —some professional, some lay—were raised to urge civilized man to get the fibre back into his diet, beginning with his daily bread. They were either ignored or reviled.

It was not until 1980 that the Royal College of Physicians published, at long last, a report giving some recognition to the place of fibre in the diet. Even so, it was insisted that any changes towards what had been obvious to the few for so long must be tentative. There had to be escape clauses for the salvaging of professional reputations in case it all turned out to be wrong! The wording even suggested that before any detailed dietary recommendations were made to the public, prolonged clinical trials were desirable—some of which, it was admitted, might be exceedingly difficult (if not impossible) to carry out.

Incredibly, on page 105, the report makes what must be one of the most deferential understatements of all time: 'Communities subsisting on a high fibre diet are said to be less prone to constipation.' Certainly the world of science and the world of common sense are worlds apart.

This long delay over many decades awaiting the official backing to restore at least some lost fibre in our diet, is an example of incredible and inexcusable observational blindness, contributing to the prolongation of preventable grievous bodily harm to millions. Belatedly now, the Health Education Council (HEC) recommends that we should eat, on average, at least one-third more dietary fibre than we do. At the same time, in order to secure the co-operation of the baking industries in reducing the salt content of bread, the HEC is (at the time of writing) allowing its logo and the slogan 'Bread is good for you!' to appear on the wrappers of all bread—including white bread! This is regrettable since there are no adequate grounds for proclaiming that white bread is good for anyone other than the starving who require first-aid sustenance. As well as lacking many nutrients it is lamentably low on dietary fibre.

I very much resist the current in-phrase 'high-fibre diet'. This suggests that the prevailing diet in the community is a normal-fibre diet, which it is not. Rather, let us expose the latter for what it is—a low-fibre diet by default. Only when we break away from it can we use the term 'normal-fibre diet'. Meanwhile, even if we follow the official HEC advice, we are likely to be having no more than a quarter of the fibre taken by those native Africans who are so much less prone to our Western diseases.

More unheeded evidence

Incredibly ignored has been the observational evidence of a

community's daily food in relation to its state of health. Wherever exceptionally healthy people are found, there also is a simple and consistent eating habit of whole, fresh, unrefined food. This is not to say—as the mockers like to claim—that the responsible food reformers would have us, in late twentieth-century Western culture, return to a primitive diet. But it is to say that we can gain much by searching out the essentials of the health-giving principles of primitive diets.

What we find is that communities can stay healthy on quite a small variety of locally available food, provided it is fresh and includes a proportion of the raw and uncooked. From race to race the few groups of foods enjoyed will vary tremendously. They will usually include several from the following: cereals, nuts, oil from nuts and seeds, fruit, leaf and root vegetables, herbs, growing tips of vegetation, milk, cream, butter, cheese, yoghurt, eggs, fish, fish oil and meat. By no means all of these are inclusively necessary for a healthy diet.

Searching for healthy communities, as recently as the thirties, Weston Price was able to identify, study and photograph at least fifteen remarkable examples worldwide. We take just one by way of illustration: Gaelics living in the islands of the Outer Hebrides exhibiting fine wide faces, splendid physique, superb teeth into old age, resistance to infection, rugged endurance and strength of character; notably a God-fearing and caring Christian community. Yet, in their conditions of living, everything would seem to be against them—an appalling, windswept, gale-ridden climate with minimal sunshine, frugal soil from which crops of any kind were extracted with the greatest difficulty, scanty livestock and small cottages—so called 'black houses' as they were smoke-ridden with peat fumes during both winter and summer.

There was only one source from which they could possibly derive their health—their basic food; fish, oat cakes, porridge and occasional vegetables. On some of the islands they were even without milk or dairy products.

In sharp contrast, and more revealing than any double-blind controlled trial, were simultaneous examples of Gaelics from the same stock living in the port of Stornoway on Lewis. They had a poor physique, narrow faces, and rampant dental decay. They enjoyed better housing and more modern amenities. The crucial matter was their diet. They were on the trade route of commercial food—freely available was imported angel cake, the whitest of white bread, canned marmalade, canned vegetables, canned meat, sweetened fruit juices, jams and sugar-laden confectionary of all kinds.

The food and condition of the modernized Gaelics is remarkably like the present day description of the poor state of health of mainland Scots living in the lovely fertile Highland valley, embraced by the practice of that most observant of general practitioners, Dr Walter Yellowlees (see chapter 12).

So we see the contrasting circumstances conducive to health and disease. A few and widely differing whole and fresh foods are sufficient to maintain health in almost any part of the globe. The same few commercial, depleted foods invariably undermine previously robust health when introduced.

Thousands more scientific papers dealing with suspected deficiencies have been published since my sideways look some thirty-five years ago. Volumes have been written describing the manifestations of the resultant diseases. Theses have been submitted and reputations made on the elucidation of a thousand and one deficiency diseases which need never arise. Whole new specialities have been established. What continues to defy understanding is why, in consideration of all the collective evidence across the board, the consensus voice of the health professions failed to cry out years ago, with authority, the sorely-needed message to a longsuffering public: 'You are what you eat—see to it that a good part of your daily food is as whole, fresh and unprocessed as possible.'

Light at the end of the tunnel

There is now, at last, some movement in this direction. The British Medical Association is addressing itself to putting over the constitution of a healthy diet to the public (see postscript at the end of this chapter). The Health Education Council is at least abreast of the consensus of professional opinion, such as it is. America remains five to ten years ahead of the UK in public, professional and commercial acceptance of the need for sustained dietary change—at least concerning restraint on sugar and salt consumption, reduction in total fat, recognition of the value of wholegrain cereals and co-operation of the meat, dairy and supermarket industries. There is, moreover, a sense of permanence in the changes being made, unlike Britain where there are dragging feet and a thinly disguised hope on the part of some that the food and health lobby will be a nine days' wonder and go away!

Changes of emphasis there may be, but food reform will most definitely not go away now. To their credit, several of our major food purveyors are already making radical changes, including more intelligible labelling of food content.

Yes but . . .

What about all the tremendous advances in medicine and treatment over the past hundred years? Was it not the case that half the children born in Victorian times failed to survive to adult life, and that for those who did, life expectation was scarcely more than forty years? So many of genius and talent died young, even those who were experts in the culinary art—Mrs Beeton died at the tender age of twenty-nine!

Old diseases vanquished

Nothing I have said detracts from the tremendous achievements of our times. Public health measures, including those already set out in the law of Moses, assisted by better economic conditions and protective immunization, have broken the back of great killer diseases like cholera, typhoid fever, dysentery, diphtheria and tuberculosis. Most babies and children now survive until old age.

It must be admitted that even the orthodox teaching in

favour of a wider variety of foods played a part. The poor nutrition of the industrial revolution was primarily due to insufficient quantity. To the near starving even deplete food is medicine—a situation sadly encountered in the Third World today.

New disease patterns

The faulty nutrition of today is not one of insufficient quantity. In many respects it is now of over-consumption. The worst impact of today's deplete food will be upon the new generations in the second half of life. There are many more yet to be affected. Some diseases like coronary heart disease were relatively unknown in the first quarter of this century.

Today's afflictions, such as diabetes, coronary heart disease, cancer and dementia mostly take many years to become established. They have an incubation period, but of a very different duration from those relating to the infectious diseases. It is entirely predictable that a bottle-fed baby, having sugared cows' milk and refined starch cereal, is setting out on an incubation period to a destination of disease—but precisely where may not emerge for fifty years.

Some twenty years ago, after hammering away at the *Family Doctor* magazine of the British Medical Association for failing sufficiently to promote healthy eating, I was given the opportunity to contribute an article: 'Do coronaries begin in the classroom?' I responded and was able to make the point that the seeds of the disease are sown much earlier than the classroom and are already germinating in the cradle.

Original concept of a master-disease

Through painstaking observations and deduction, Surgeon Captain T.L. Cleave linked the worst manifestations of the refinement and over-consumption of Western food to a number of the most serious degenerative diseases afflicting mankind. Among such he included: diabetes, obesity, coronary heart disease, varicose veins, deep vein thrombosis, haemorrhoids, dental disease, peptic ulcer, diverticular disease, cancer of the bowel, and toxaemia of pregnancy. All these and more he saw as manifestations of a single underlying master-disease to which he designated the term 'Saccharine Disease' (related to sugar). The mechanisms giving rise to these disease manifestations were: removal of fibre and protein by refinement of food, and over-consumption facilitated by concentrated bulk-free food.

These concepts, which Cleave began to advance in the mid-fifties, were so revolutionary to the orthodox that it was inevitable he would initially suffer the reaction which has greeted so many of the great reformers in the history of medicine: indifference, disbelief, hostility and ridicule. It has been bad enough for pioneers who seek to upturn established belief in the cause and treatment of just one disease. Here was a relatively unknown man claiming to have discovered the underlying cause of the majority of the degenerative diseases of our time, ranging from such unlikely bedfellows as dental caries and diabetes. Preposterous!

This man had the nerve to propound that they were not separate diseases but all manifestations of a single master-disease. The total package was altogether too much to swallow. But parts of it soon began to find commendation from the not inconsiderable number of lay and professional people, who were convinced through observation alone of the damaging consequences to health of modern sophisticated food, without hitherto having fully understood the mechanism. One facet of his work was relatively easily proved in practice—that which stemmed from his use of simple miller's bran to prevent and relieve the disabling constipation which beset the wartime Royal Navy, deprived of fresh vegetables and fibre. So much so, that by the sixties he had become known to a wider public as 'the bran man'. Eventually, the dietary fibre aspects of his work caught on to such an extent that his even more important exposure of the consequences of over-consumption facilitated by refined foods, and sugar in particular, continued to be neglected. Although his saccharine or master-disease concept had not yet found ready understanding, nobody was laughing by the end of his days in 1983. He lived to see the essence of his work vindicated.

Fortunately for those of us whose prime concern is getting an effective message over to the public, the question as to whether a disease is but a manifestation of a comprehensive master-disease or is a separate disease sharing a common underlying cause is of little consequence. What matters, in the interests of prevention and treatment, is the recognition of the factor that is common to both cases: deplete food.

Much as I feel that the whole of Cleave's brilliant and logical concept will eventually be validated, I fear that to insist upon it now may be to hinder the interests of health education. The health professions are trained up in the fragmentary study of individual diseases. Although they may now be ready to acknowledge impoverished nutrition as the major underlying cause of a number of separate diseases, they are not yet ready to concede that these diseases are merely manifestations of one major somatic disease.

Rather than pursuing this apparently unfruitful argument, it is much more apt to consider the wider ramifications of the underlying cause, hinted at by Dr Miles Robinson in his introduction to the American edition of Cleave's book; this is, the consequence of the removal of vitamins and other nutrients in the refining processes. Cleave graciously refers to my repeated discussions with him on these matters in his concluding chapter. He told me that it would take all of his lifetime and effort to put over the central part of his message—and it did! He would leave it to others to enlarge on the matter of vital substances and trace elements.

This, in all humility, is part of what I seek to do in this book in order that in choosing health, daily food may not only be largely unrefined, unsophisticated and free from excesses of sugary matter, but also whole, live and fresh. To this end, I nominate complete food as the handmaid of positive health and deplete food as the big brother of ill health.

Preventable deterioration of brain and body

One vital group of substances is at the very heart of the fat/cholesterol controversy. I refer to essential fatty acids (EFA) which are deficient in deplete food. These substances have been called structural fats and appear to be important in the development of the structure of brain and nerve conductors.

One can almost predict that there will arise a number of 'mystery' diseases stemming from a deficiency of some EFA-like substance and trace minerals governing the delicate electrical functions between nerves and muscles.

Like the case of Annie.

Dementia in the making

Annie was sixty-two, lived alone and had been widowed for fourteen years. She never had much idea about wholefood or live food when her husband was alive, but she did at least produce something like meat and cooked vegetables and a pudding on most days. After his death Annie lost interest, and the quality and even the quantity of her daily food progressively deteriorated. Eventually, it centred around the teapot, biscuits, white bread, confectioner's cake and an occasional meat pie.

Even before the age of sixty her mind was failing. She became increasingly forgetful, agitated, anti-social and cussid! She was the despair of her few remaining relatives, the neighbours, the health visitors and her general practitioner. Mounting concern about her self-neglect, stench and squalor in her little home and the ever-present ominous smell of paraffin, led to a medical consultant in diseases of the elderly being called in. He reported to the GP that she was suffering from episodes of confusion. He noted fissuring and cracking at the angles of the mouth, also rawness of the tongue, with haemorrhages beneath. He had no doubt in identifying nutritional deficiency of at least the B and C vitamins and iron. He offered her a short spell in hospital to build her up but she adamantly refused. He finally prescribed vitamin and iron injections by the district nurse, meals-on-wheels and a home help.

She subsequently resisted all these ministrations and some months later was admitted to hospital in emergency with acute abdominal pain, bowel obstruction, distended bladder and total confusion. She improved somewhat, but demanded to be allowed home after a few weeks. Back in the same conditions she soon deteriorated. A few months later—with the neighbours up in arms—she was removed compulsorily to hospital on a doctor's and magistrate's order, and died shortly afterwards.

Annie was a sad example of Deplete Food Disease of the elderly. Ignorance and self-neglect were major factors, as they are in the thousands of similar cases occurring all the time. Confusion, mania and depression in these cases are the continuing despair of relatives and neighbours which spills over as illness, stress and unfounded guilt in others. Even worse than all these is the alarming increase of the more fully developed condition Alzheimer's disease, or pre-senile dementia.

Official medical opinion does not yet admit to a known cause of this disease. Speculation is not encouraged in the medical profession. Yet, if we consider the precise balance of the tissue fluids, salts, minerals and trace elements necessary to ensure that the delicate electrical responses take place at the nerve junctions, and if we reflect how many of these vital substances are missing from a diet like Annie's, can we really be surprised when the brain fails to work adequately or that degenerative disease of the brain occurs?

I predict, for instance, that in due course the greater number of cases of multiple sclerosis, myasthenia gravis, the muscular dystrophies, Parkinson's disease and pre-senile dementia will be classified as Deplete Food Disease, or whatever term for this underlying cause is eventually adopted. If slow-acting viruses turn out to be implicated in Alzheimer's disease, or other diseases of nerve and/or muscle tissue, I will not be regarding the virus as the underlying cause, merely the invader into the seedbed of ill-health and a consequent triggering or aggravating factor.

Cancer and carcinogens—underlying cause or trigger factor?

Circumstances in the environment known to be linked with cancer, such as asbestos, tobacco smoke, tar, nitrates and x-rays are referred to as 'carcinogens'. Some descriptions suggest that they cause or produce cancer, but do they?

I prefer to believe that the underlying cause of cancer is to be found in the seedbed of the body cells. If those cells are deficient in vital protective substances, then any one of the numerous insults to our tissues with which we have to live in civilized society year after year will be liable to trigger off cancer, sometimes in more than one site simultaneously.

Cancer is always liable to arise whenever the body's precious immune system is impaired so that its ability to recognize, kill or reject foreign substances or cells is diminished. When this happens, the cell regeneration systems have become overtaxed by being deprived of some of the essential repair materials.

The experts are all too ready to remind us that nearly all diseases are multi-factorial in origin, that is, several causes contribute to the condition. This, of course, is evident in the case of cancer, but it must not deter me from stating that, in my opinion, by far and away the most important factor leading to the onset of cancer is deplete nutrition. If I were to point to just one general observation which substantiates this claim, it would be that the basis of non-orthodox physical measures which can sometimes successfully reverse the cancer process nearly always includes live, whole food. Attitudes of mind are also important, but secondary to a healing diet. It is axiomatic that if right food can achieve the reversal of a disease as inexorable as cancer, right food adopted soon enough is the most effective single means of preventing it.

I am aware that this is a simplification of a highly complex subject. A tremendous amount of work over generations has been done on cancer cells, immunity, genes and factors which can alter genes, for which we must be grateful, but health education advice in regard to keeping our resistance in peak condition is painfully slow to emerge.

Deplete food is likely to increase the cancer risk in all tissues of the body, but there is one location especially where depletion will have an effect. That place is the large bowel—the colon and rectum. It is, in the West, the commonest form of cancer apart from that of the lung, where tobacco is the major triggering factor. Studies of races where incidence is low, all point to fibre in the diet as being the critical factor. The toxic breakdown products of the small, hard stools formed by the refined foods of Western society have slow and prolonged contact with the bowel walls. The longer this goes on—and it can be fifty years or more before the cells rebel—the greater the liability to bowel cancer. More happily, insufficient dietary fibre is one of the easiest of the depletions to make good. Simple miller's bran and change of dietary habit can at least prevent any further damage, if not necessarily the consequences of a lifetime of wrong habit. There is now the emerging likelihood that the wonderful ability of dietary fibre to absorb toxic substances may also help to protect against cancer in other sites of the body. But there are other deficiencies in our food which need to be restored—not just fibre. Protection requires the whole gamut of vital substances in live food.

Cancer—avoidance of trigger factors

It is difficult to refer to the hundreds of substances and influences in civilized society which can serve as triggers to cancer, without provoking that very anxiety which I am at pains to avoid. It has to be remembered that for most cancers the provocation is one that has been repeated many times, over many years (though there are exceptions, like asbestos or large-dose radiation, where short exposure can provoke early cancer). But, as with the legions of germs in our environment, we cannot eliminate them all, or avoid contact with them.

Avoidance of cancer is achieved by keeping our personal defences intact, and the first priority in doing that is the adequate nourishment of these immune and defence systems by complete nutrition.

Secondary defence is prudent avoidance of such things as lead, asbestos, formaldehyde, herbicides, smoke, moulds, and pesticide residues. Avoid unnecessary x-ray examinations. You are the one most likely to know how many you have had during your lifetime. Also important is the avoidance of prolonged use of drugs, unless deemed essential. On the food front, we need to go very sparingly on processed oils and fats; to avoid rancid fat of any kind; not to reheat fat more than once for frying or roasting; and to avoid any foods afflicted with mould, including sadly the frequent consumption of some popular cheeses where mould is encouraged to enhance flavour.

The way of health

These are some of the hazards to be avoided so far as is possible. There are many foods left to choose from which are whole and delicious. They are further detailed in chapter 6.

Postscript

The British Medical Association has at last seen the light. In a report entitled 'Diet, Nutrition and Health' dated 1986 a scientific committee has formulated Dietary Objectives for the nation. Their recommendations include a reduction in total fat, a reduction of sugar and salt intake and an increase in dietary fibre. It is with much satisfaction that I note that whole grain products are advocated, as opposed to products to which bran and other fibre has been added. They make the point that using the whole grain product will ensure increased intake of minerals, trace elements and other micronutrients.

Most intriguingly the authors of the report are at particular pains to defend themselves against possible cricitism for making recommendations unsupported by scientific evidence.

With what immense pleasure would Allinson and Arbuthnot Lane have read this report!

☆　　☆　　☆

Nutrition is the basis of defence against cancer—beginning in the soil.

ANDRÉ VOISIN (1959)

REFERENCE

Geoffrey Cannon, Caroline Walker, 'Just How Well Do We Eat?' *(Observer* Jan 27th 1985).

Geoffrey Cannon, Caroline Walker, *The Food Scandal* (Century 1984).

Kenneth Vickery, 'Healthy Food for Thought' (*Observer* Feb 3rd 1985).

Kenneth Vickery, 'Positive Health and the Relationship of Man to His Living Environment' (*Royal Sanitary Institute* May 3rd 1953).

Royal College of Physicians London, 'Smoking and Health' First Report 1962.

Royal College of Physicians London, *Medical Aspects of Dietary Fibre* (Pitman Medical 1980).

Weston A. Price, *Nutrition and Physical Degeneration* (American Academy of Applied Nutrition 1948).

Kenneth Vickery, 'Do Coronaries Begin in the Classroom?' (BMA *Family Doctor* Sep 1965).

T.L. Cleave, *The Saccharine Disease* (Wright Bristol 1974, Keats Publishing USA 1975).

3
Genesis of Depletion

How come, then, this depletion which is at the root of so much disease? We need to follow the causes right from the source of all nutriment—which is in the soil—along the highways of commerce, to the food which is ready for eating.

Impoverished soil—ignorant neglect

Life depends on a flow of nutrients from the soil—either through vegetation to man direct, or through animal and thence to man. The storehouse of life is the living soil which is formed by the constant erosion of mineral rock together with the broken-down fabric of returned organic matter. The elements essential for life are widely distributed across the face of the earth and in the rivers and seas.

We can thus visualize an ascending and dynamic food chain within a cycle of life and decay. The greatest single cause of disease in plant, animal or man is some depletion of this food chain or man-made interference with this cycle of life.

Left to itself, nature ensures that all organic waste returns to the soil. It is only man who takes, without returning, as though there were no tomorrow, and who thereby compounds the most fundamental cause of disease in the plants and animals in his charge, resulting in his own ill health. For the fact is that an adequate intake of the minerals and living wealth of the soil is an essential foundation of health. These

47

are required for elaboration in the healthy plant to the form required by man. It may be that the resultant vegetation will be assimilated by an animal, similarly dependent for health on a healthy soil, and will in turn be eaten by man. Unhealthy crops and unhealthy animals inevitably predispose disease in man. There is nothing fanciful in the headline: 'Farming Can Seriously Damage Your Health.'

Good husbandry in accordance with nature's principles was the order of the day among responsible farmers and gardeners until the mid-nineteenth century. Then almost overnight many thought they had discovered the panacea and royal road to perpetual fertility from a sack.

Utopia with a backlash

Spurred by the industrial population explosion, man found that he could achieve a dramatic increase in crop yield by the application of compounds of nitrogen, phosphorus and potassium in crude chemical form. He found blessed relief from the heavy chore of muck spreading. And there seemed no need for all the time and effort of animal husbandry, if arable farming was his choice. The age of monoculture had arrived. There appeared no end to the potential of fertility by artificial means. The old curse upon Adam of sweat and toil was surely now overcome?

What was not appreciated was that this honeymoon of crop fertility was only possible by dint of previous centuries of arduous husbandry when as much as was taken, and more, was put back into the soil. As human waste has been channelled into water carriage sewage systems (a necessary expedient) and farm animals have been replaced by tractors and straw burning prevails, so now there is an increasing lack of humus being returned to the soil. The balance of the soil is upset. The big visible indicator of the soil organisms, the earthworm, disappears. Crop disease becomes rampant.

In the early years of artificial fertilization relatively simple pesticides were effective. With each succeeding crop generation the organisms of disease become more resistant, and new and more devastating pesticides are resorted to. We now have the situation where pesticides with the lethal potential of methylisocyanate (Bhopal) are deemed necessary, worldwide, to combat disease.

Soil abuse—an incubation period

Intriguingly, and in further confirmation of the application of similar simple principles throughout nature, there is in the case of the living organism which is the soil an incubation period before the worst consequences of abuse come home to roost—just as in human disease. Given a previously good fertile soil this period of grace can be a hundred years or more.

But the soil has now rebelled to such an extent, and so obviously, that even the most orthodox of gardeners and farmers are being compelled to consider ways and means of organic return. They see that for artificial fertilizers to continue to be effective there must be a simultaneous return of organic matter.

So now in the eighties most of the TV and radio pundits of gardening hold forth about the merits of humus and the compost heap as though this has always been received knowledge. Gardeners with longer memories recall that no more than twenty years ago the advocates of composting were liable to the same ridicule as the proponents of wholemeal bread, and that tiny minority of enlightened farmers were dubbed 'disciples of muck and magic' because they were prepared to labour harder for less profit to put organic heart back into the land. Thankfully their numbers are steadily increasing.

The leaching of the land

From the time that man moved forward from being a hunter/gatherer to a husbandman he has been liable to take more out of the land than he returned and to cut down more trees than he planted. When the world population was small this may not have been too serious. Even so, man's activities 2,000 and more years ago around the Mediterranean basin had already spawned vast deserts, formerly the granaries of ancient empires.

The really critical time is now—late twentieth century. The world population is exploding at an alarming rate. Demands for food production on the precious few inches of topsoil the world over are intensifying. Forests and trees everywhere, despite their importance in atmospheric renewal, are being used up relentlessly. Constantly, as indeed from the dawn of time, there is the washing out of land fertility as minerals in the soil are carried down to the sea—adding to its abundance of latent fertility. This leaching process is intensified wherever land is badly managed and humus content becomes low. Leaching of added chemical fertilizers is liable to be rapid, wasteful and expensive.

Given millions of years, geological movement causes sea-beds to become land and land to become the floor of the sea, and in this way the whole process of renewed land fertility begins again. But this slow process will not save today's teeming millions. There are probably more people alive now on the face of the earth than have in total lived throughout previous recorded history. Unless we are prepared to undertake the painstaking and labour-intensive efforts of restoring all organic waste to the land, all grown food will become progressively more deplete. Crops will become more and more deficient in the minerals and traces which are not provided in the sacks of crude nitrogen, phosphate and potassium fertilizers. Ways of restoring trace elements to the soil must be found. Radical reform of land and resource management is urgent and imperative. (See chapter 13.)

Depletion in the factory farm

Few farmers or veterinary surgeons would now deny that a large part of the disease encountered in livestock is connected with deficiency of vital substance and mineral in soil and vegetation. These deficiencies are further compounded by factory farming of livestock. Without resort to antibiotics and other medicinal drugs, intensive animal husbandry would rapidly collapse. A ready illustration of the deprived consequences of farm factory food is to be seen in the bones of some broiler chickens. Spontaneous fractures abound and the difference in strength of the skeleton in comparison with a free-range bird is obvious. A useful source of cheap protein for many, but hardly the stuff for sustaining the health of man. Sad to note also that not even healthy-looking farmed fish are immune to the diseases of civilization. It was noticed some years ago that 60% or more of farmed rainbow trout in the United States had cancer of the liver, which is very rare in wild trout. A controlled investigation pointed strongly to a commercial dry feed made from cottonseed meal and fishmeal with additives.

Storage and transport

No small part of the inflictions suffered by food arise from the need to prevent spoilage during transport and storage. It is an inconvenient fact that the more life and vitality contained in a foodstuff, the more liable it will be to fermentation, oxidation, mould, infestation and deterioration generally.

Beyond the farm gate

In the interests of easy availability of bulk food for the masses, there is liable to be progressive affliction of already deprived food all the way from the farm to the dinner table.

Refinement

The single most damaging and depriving consequence to health arises from refinement and concentration of the starchy and sugary content of cereal and root crops. The foremost purpose of this activity is to produce highly calorific foods which can be transported with a minimum of bulk and which will not go bad in storage. A secondary purpose is to satisfy mankind's addiction to sweet foods and our alleged public preference to white bread and other white-flour products.

Heat treatment

Storage and preservation is also a motive for that great range of food processing involving heat treatment, such as canning and commercial cooking. This also involves considerable loss of vital substances.

The cooking of food has enabled man to enlarge his choice, particularly with meat, fish, legumes and root vegetables. He has adapted to eating a proportion of heat-treated food over many thousands of years. Indeed in today's world certain foods, if they are to be taken at all, require heat treatment for safety reasons. This will include all meats and milk.

Refrigeration

A considerable twentieth-century boon to the conservation and preservation of food supply is refrigeration and deep freezing. The loss of vitality to food can be very little and it has enabled the superseding of canning, dehydration, salting and smoking.

Irradiation

The bombardment of food with gamma rays is a method of food preservation which has been undergoing several years' active investigation. The trials have shown promising results and no significant hazards to health have emerged. The radiation behaves rather like sunlight and interacts with the bacteria which cause food spoilage. Harmful bacteria are also subdued. Risks of food poisoning can be reduced and the process is found particularly good for foods otherwise eaten raw such as the roll mop herring, smoked salmon and spices.

Certainly the early results are promising and this method of preservation seems better than the chemical alternative. The worst effects of overtreatment appear to be upon taste and flavour. The only nagging doubt is the possibility of causing mischievous mutations in bacteria. Public reaction may be anticipated from a vocal minority opposed to the extension of use of any form of nuclear energy.

Institutional food—the great British disaster

It is sad enough when, as a result of misleading reassurance, ignorance or indifference, we inflict deprived food upon ourselves. It is even sadder when we visit it upon others. Most inexcusably perhaps in hospitals. Yet only a very few enlightened hospitals have made any serious attempt to break away from serving the same deplete food which was partly to blame for the patients being in hospital in the first place. Instead of being regarded as a healing and educative opportunity, food is moved even further away from the health professionals. Dietitians have had little say in its overall provision. The catering managers are now being styled 'hotel-services managers' and ward domestics have now taken over from nurses the responsibility of dealing with patients in their daily selection from the menu.

Those responsible for provisions in canteens and residential establishments carry a heavy responsibility. This will include managers of schools and colleges, keepers of nursing and residential homes, catering managers, and prison governors. Observations made on recent informal visits suggest that enlightenment, although increasing slightly, remains at a very low ebb. A major problem is the established food habits and the resistance to change. Cost is another ever-present hindrance to the better integrity of food.

It is exceptional to find in any institution that wholemeal bread is the norm provided. At best some inferior kind of 'brown' bread is available as an alternative to squares of sliced white. Cakes and biscuits are a common feature in the daily diet and are usually all made with white flour. Sugar in its various forms is also liberally provided. Hundreds of thousands of gallons of sweetened custard are daily poured onto already sweetened puddings and pastries made with the crudest of refined flour. Millions of hamburgers oozing with dubious fat, sandwiched between lifeless carbohydrate baps, are daily grabbed by hungry youngsters.

A typical institutional breakfast, unless special request is made, begins with proprietary cereals of the cornflake type, usually not wholegrain, already sweetened and taken with added sugar. This is often followed by bacon or sausage and fried white bread, and concluded with white toast, butter and highly-sugared marmalade together with sweetened beverages.

There will be meat courses for one or both of the remaining main meals accompanied by well-cooked cabbage or similar vegetable, liberally salted. Such a diet, day after day with little or no opportunity for fresh fruit and salad, is an almost certain recipe for ill-health, sooner or later. For most residents some degree of constipation may be anticipated.

A particular responsibility rests where the inmates are long-term captives. This will apply to long-stay hospitals, including those for the mentally ill or subnormal. Prisons, borstals and corrective youth centres are obvious examples. It has been a repeated observation that the demeanour, state of restlessness or otherwise, aggression or tranquillity of residents is very closely related to the quality of the food. Particularly important is a sufficient daily intake of the water-soluble B vitamins and dietary fibre.

The infliction, for instance, of constipation upon service men or prisoners in confined conditions, amounts to cruelty. Many have a very limited time available to go to the toilet and what they do have is often aggravated by a sense of haste and lack of privacy. Children in hostels and boarding schools may similarly suffer. There is no sadder sight to my mind than the well-meaning gift of an enormous iced and sugar-laden birthday or Christmas cake, generously donated or passed on to the local children's home or hospital. We really have no excuse for such folly and ignorance.

Will they never learn?

I have never ceased to be amazed over the years, when illness surfaces and demands attention, how little interest is shown by the hospital team in the living habits of the patient. Patients admitted to hospital for operation are likely to be provided with skilled and superb treatment and then allowed to lapse back into the same habits and circumstances which caused or contributed to their illness in the first place.

Healing against the odds

Repair and healing of damaged tissues at the best of times draws heavily upon the body's supply and store of such vital substances as the A, B, C and K vitamins. The demands following major heart surgery and organ transplant are prodigious.

One would expect during the early days of heart, liver and other major organ transplants that the surgical team would leave no stone unturned to ensure that the extensive healing process got off to the best possible start. One would anticipate that at least for some weeks before and after the operation patients would be expected to co-operate in the best of whole-food healing diets.

It was so sad therefore that within a matter of days of one of the first ever heart and lung transplants, the hospital spokesman facing the world's press was at such pains to emphasize the normality of the child patient's recovery that he told us she had had fish and chips for lunch!

Published accounts in regard to some heart transplant cases suggest that in view of the presumed need to safeguard against infection, all food in the post-operative period is heat sterilized. In one classic case the food consisted of reconstituted dried egg, scrambled, together with tinned fruit (doubtless laden with sugar). One patient pleading monotony was allowed to add bottled sauce to the egg. A patient after discharge rejected a relative's attempts to provide him with a calorie-controlled, low-cholesterol meal and opted for fish and chips. He also made a conscious decision to continue smoking.

I find no evidence (unless it is happening very recently) that patients undergoing major surgery or organ transplant are advised in the matter of a wholefood healing diet. We can surely at long last now anticipate that priority in future may be given to patients who are prepared to co-operate in at least the rudiments of the official advice now spelt out in *Eating for a Healthier Heart*.

And now pacemakers for dogs

I doubt if any authentic case has ever been demonstrated of an animal in its fully natural, wild conditions suffering coronary thrombosis. But animals share many of man's afflictions when they come to live with him and become part of his food habits —and by all accounts long before old age.

A Golden Retriever, described in a press report as young, was said to have suffered three 'coronaries' in one day. To the delight of the owner, the dog was able to have the implant of a second-hand pacemaker, and is said to be back to his old exuberant self. The report does not mention if the owner is considering whether the household food may be responsible for the dog's degenerative disease.

'Ask of the beasts and they shall teach thee'

I am indebted to the captive and domesticated animal for much of the early circumstantial evidence providing the encouragement to persevere with man and his food.

In pursuit of excellence and profit, those responsible for the rearing of animals have come to pay more attention to their food than man does to his. I noted in the early fifties that certain continental race-horse breeders rediscovered that stamina and form was related to the quality of the feed. And the winning fodder turned out to be organically grown.

We should probably have had to suffer much longer with the agene bleaching of bread had it not been for the commercial interests of dog breeders. Hysteria in dogs was firmly linked with the nerve-poisoning effects of food made from agenized white flour. Not only was care taken that dogs were no longer fed agene, it also became standard practice that the greater part of all cereal used for dog feeds contained some or all of the germ and roughage of the cereal.

In 1959 a TV programme referred to the considerable success at the Bristol, Clifton and West of England Zoo in what then was the very difficult feat of breeding gorillas in captivity. It was stated that the breakthrough had only come following a most careful review of the diet of the parents and offspring— the mainstay of which was now fresh fruit and vegetables and specially made wholemeal bread.

On further enquiry I received a most helpful reply from the Director/Superintendent confirming the diet and noting also that vitamin and mineral supplement was given daily together with thyroid extract. I am particularly intrigued to note that the motto under the Society's heraldic crest bears the inscription: 'Ask of the Beasts and they shall teach thee.' I find this is derived from the book of Job (chapter 12, verse 7).

The end of the line—deplete food for many

Returning to man, it is all too easy to see how enormous quantities of deprived, lifeless, sophisticated food reach the consumer following one depletion after another.

The food technologists are faced with two apparently contradictory trends: people want convenience foods, but now they also want the food to be fresher and healthier. All too often it will only appear to be more fresh. Meanwhile hamburgers, chips, sugar-laden confections and sweetened drinks, together with a multi-million pound snacks industry, continue to be the mainstay of millions when away from home.

It is sadly all too easy to see how unthinking man can incur, through his food, an increasing debt of vital protective substances. The wonder is not that Deplete Food Disease is common including the so-called mystery diseases of nerve and muscle function, but that we are not overwhelmed by it.

☆   ☆   ☆

Soil science is the foundation of protective medicine.

ANDRÉ VOISIN.

☆   ☆   ☆

A farmer should farm as if he were going to live forever and live as if he were going to die tomorrow.

Old Farming Axiom.

REFERENCE

André Voisin, *Soil, Grass and Cancer* (Crosby Lockwood 1959).

'Liver Cancer in Farmed Rainbow Trout' (*New Scientist* No. 306 Sep 27th 1960).

Eating for a Healthier Heart (Health Education Council 1985).

4
Health by Design

We have arrived at a point in this exposure of so much that is wrong where some form of encouragement must be delayed no further.

The good news is that disease and ill-health are not the inevitable lot of man. We have the means at our disposal to attain a far better level of health than is currently enjoyed or endured by many. For those not yet on their way to better health, this can be secured by the adoption of relatively simple —and certainly not burdensome—changes in daily habits of living. Yes, we ourselves can do something about it, and the more people around us who do likewise, the better for all. The degree of potential improvement is, of course, dependent upon our condition and age when we start to make the changes.

What is health?

So far we have confined ourselves to the shortest of definitions —wholeness. There are many more, all of them longer. Lord Horder gave much thought to definition when writing *Health and a Day* and concluded that, while the healthy state may be described, it is almost impossible to define. We owe to him the perception that health is something much more positive than a mere absence of disease. Not for Lord Horder the idealistic delusion of the founders of the British National Health Service that if only enough facilities are provided for everyone to be treated, only health will remain!

One reason for the difficulty in defining health is that it is not a fixed state. It is dynamic, responsive and ever-changing. Furthermore, the health of an organism can be adequately considered only in relation to the health of surrounding species. In other words, ecological health. Having said this, the fact is that we all know what our expectations of health are in terms of vitality, brightness of eye, mental vigour, appetite, weight, sleep and general well-being—all so disappointingly fulfilled for many.

Health by design

We are designed to be in health. All living organisms are equipped with wonderful powers of resistance to the continual and ongoing assaults to which they lay themselves open as they live and move in the hazardous world about them. This will include resistance to harmful radiation from the sun, the cosmos and from the activity of man; to all the many insects, microbes and viruses which abound in nature; to the many physical and chemical inflictions upon body cells. Coupled with resistance are the built-in, automatically induced and constant healing processes; the almost instantaneous ones, like the gobbling up of germs in our tissues and bloodstream by mobile, scavenging cells; the blood clotting, and the longer term ones like the healing of wounds and broken bones. Some species can even grow new limbs and parts to replace lost and injured ones.

If these precious systems are in full working order, we stay in health. But, increasingly in today's overcrowded and hectic world, these systems of defence and repair are deficient or overloaded and disease takes hold. There are very definite reasons why this is happening. Disease does not just happen out of the blue. Disease is a consequence. Somewhere along the line there has been default.

Disease by default

The fact is, to manufacture and maintain the biological systems of body structure, cell resistance and repair, there is required throughout life a flow of nourishing foodstuff, which includes whole and live food factors containing vitamins and the major and trace minerals. When these are deficient, as they frequently are, disease can and does take hold. Deplete food is therefore the central underlying cause of nurtural disease. To be more specific, the exquisite materials required to build up the resistance and healing factors are not to be found in junk food, such as hamburgers, ice-cream, confectionery, chips and cola! Alongside this cause there are a number of other influences which are only worthy of the term 'contributing factors'. These include climate, microbes, radiation, chemicals and the influence of the mind.

Never again

I feel it necessary to justify myself for going on at length about consequences of depletion, and for repeating the concept in differing context throughout the book. I am earnestly asking that the momentum of the interest in food and health be maintained so that we get to the heart of the matter of wholeness. It must not stop short at negative advice on sugar and salt, or positive advice on wholegrain and dietary fibre. Above all, it must not get bogged down in the complexity of fats. Never again must inappropriate demands of statistical scientific methods be allowed to hinder the demonstrably best interests of food and health.

Deficiency—the order of the day

For optimum health of plant, animal and man, a continuing flow of a wide variety of nutrients is necessary. Alongside the well-known building blocks of carbohydrates, proteins and fats, the human system requires a wide range of vital substances and mineral elements. There is a very wide distribution on the face of the earth of the more important of these. Local deficiencies *can* occur naturally but are more often man-made.

The popular bookshelves are filled with paperbacks displaying exciting titles. Some extol the virtues of the well-known vitamins; others point to missing vital factors in the food; others deal with minerals and whole books are written about just one trace element—like selenium. Yet the standard book on home health care in the public library continues to perpetuate the orthodox received opinion that, provided 'a good mixed diet' is taken, there is no need to worry about nutritional deficiency.

Wherein lies the truth? The overwhelming balance of observational evidence is that, at a time of unprecedented world population increase, there is an accelerating decrease in the integrity of the food that enters the mouth of man.

What about genes and heredity?

There is endless speculation as to how much of disease is hereditary and how much of it due to the influences of our surroundings, including food. Cleave has performed a valuable service in pointing out how rare true hereditary defects are in nature. Extremely rare in the wild, and even in man seldom exceeding two or three cases per thousand live births for any one condition. The point which Cleave has made above all is that we have a prevalent habit of regarding more conditions as hereditary than truly are. This is undesirable. First, because it causes a sense of helplessness; and secondly, because it diverts attention from environmental factors which may be open to remedy.

We have to distinguish between diseases arising from inherited constitution and those which are termed 'congenital', i.e. they have arisen in the womb as a result of external influences—such as deplete food. During pregnancy there are very heavy demands upon vital substances to form the cells and genetic materials of the growing embryo. When we look at the deprived food of so many expectant mothers, can we really be surprised that birth defects are so uniquely prevalent in man? Hereditary disposition, however, is bound up in that perplexing variability as to whether—and if so, how early in life—we succumb to environmental causes and factors in disease. People vary markedly in susceptibility. There is the apparent unfairness that one may quickly succumb to disease through only minor departures from the laws of health, while another may break them flagrantly for a lifetime and seem to get away with it. This can be a despair to health educationists who find it very difficult to convince the public that habits of living really matter.

The factor here, and a powerful one, is our inherited make-up. This has two components—the genetic, from the genes of our parents, and the familial, which is all that part of our endowment derived after conception from the family environment. Together, these influences suggest that the length of our lives usually turns out very similar to that of our parents. But none of us can yet be sure what is our constitutional level of inherited resistance to disease. Twenty cigarettes a day can send one man to an early grave, but will scarcely affect the lifespan of another. Both, however, will stand the best possible chance if their nutrition seedbed is sound. Take no notice, therefore, of the old reprobate at the back of the hall who will boast—following the doctor's lecture—that he has broken all the rules for a lifetime! The bell will almost certainly toll much sooner for the rest of us.

Caring for ourselves

The conditional good news is that we choose health by choosing the food we were designed for. The bad news is that if we do not, disease is likely to choose us.

We are not necessarily stuck with the shape or substance of our bodies as they are now. Pictures of 'the slimmer of the year'—before and after—are enough to convince us of that.

We take heart that every one of the millions of millions of cells in our body is undergoing constant renewal—maybe a hundred or more times in a lifetime. It surely makes sense to ensure that the best possible material is continuously available through our daily food.

A measure of food reform along the lines of chapter 6 is our most tangible way of coming closer to our potential in health. Even for those with advanced chronic disease, some measure of improvement can be expected—if no more than the relief of exhausting constipation, which so easily besets the bedfast. For others, there can be a drop in the frequency and severity of epileptic fits, improvement in hyperactivity and even some relief from intractable mental illness.

So much for temporal argument in favour of health. The good news continues in the next chapter, where we see that we are not alone in wanting mankind to enjoy good health.

Some few, by endowment at birth, may seem to be unaffected by careless habits of living for a lifetime. Most others, sooner or later, succumb to the consequences.

5
Revelation of Health

The acme of the good news is that the design which carries our potential of good health is of God. We are provided with exquisite built-in systems of growth, renewal, repair and defence. As the psalmist observed, we are fearfully and wonderfully made by God who provides for our every need now and eternally. He is the source of everything we require to be in health, if only we will obey him.

'Nature with open volume stands'

This opening to the perceptive hymn by Isaac Watts (1707) reminds us that the source of a great part of the revelation of health is to be found in the open book of nature, as man observes the soil, the seed, nurture, growth, decay and new life. We marvel at the constant discoveries of nature's beautiful extravagant, randomly unlikely provisions, which are excitingly predictive—that a creature with an intellect must in time exist to observe and make use of them.

We recall the many facets of nature expressed by others over the years as we determine to work with her. Nature is the totality of what exists and the ways in which things act. Amazing wonders are discovered by simple observation. Nature admits no lie and is ignored only at a price. She confers neither rewards nor punishments—merely consequences. She is the art of God. Her potential is beautifully expressed by

Longfellow:

> And Nature, the old nurse, took
> The child upon her knee,
> Saying 'Here is a story-book
> Thy Father has written for thee.'
>
> 'Come wander with me,' she said,
> 'Into regions yet untrod;
> And read what is still unread
> In the manuscripts of God.'

The fabric of man

A most vital statement by our Maker, concerning the origin of human life and health, comes in the first pages of the Bible: 'The Lord God formed man of the dust of the ground' (Genesis 2:7). It is indeed certain that every molecule of man's body derives from the soil, the dust of the ground, in association with air and water. By a series of remarkable organic chemical combinations, assisted by sunlight, elements of the dust of the ground are elaborated into living vegetation whose leaf, root, fruit and seed becomes the food of animal and man. Almost literally, 'all flesh is grass' (Isaiah 40:6).

At the very heart of the fabric of man are those molecules of a substance known as DNA (deoxyribonucleic acid) which comprise the genes with that remarkable spiral the 'double helix'. Then we have the four kinds of chemical units in tandem pairs which in great numbers link the two sides of the double helix together. Here we have the basis of the genetic or DNA code which determines the inherited form of each of the multitude of developing organisms. This code interacts with other organic materials to form the main building-blocks of the body, the proteins in many varieties and permutations.

I mention this recently revealed wonder of biology to remind us that it can only function in perfection if a flow of the necessary vital substances elaborated from the living soil is received. Where this is deprived, for any reason, can we be surprised that cell development may be stunted and that such things as cancer and developmental deformity arise?

Dust of the earth

The dust which we are made of is held in a precious few inches of topsoil on the face of the earth. Intimately bound with the mineral elements is humus, a product of the breakdown of returned organic material. Humus is the starting point of new life, serving to hold water as a nutrient base for the seed and roots of new life and, when healthy, teeming with organisms capable of breaking down decayed, organic matter and elaborating new growth. All in the presence of essential enzymes together with air and sunlight.

Release from the rocky fabric of essential minerals and trace elements is governed by the extent of organic matter, particularly the urine and droppings of livestock. Indeed, the wonderful system of conservation and release when required can be seen as the foreknowledge of our great Creator to hold in reserve the mineral for untold aeons until stimulated by husbandry.

Can we really believe that these three major components of air so vital to life—oxygen, nitrogen and carbon dioxide—just happened by chance in such perfect proportion? Indeed, just as life is dependent on the proportion of these gases, so is the maintenance of their proportion dependent upon life. We hardly begin to fathom the length, breadth and depth of all things working together in the total ecology.

Divine ecology

We do not find the word 'ecology' in the Scriptures. It did not come into use until the late nineteenth century. Yet the whole Bible abounds in the ecological concept, with plants, animals and man in living relationship with each other and with their environment. The earth, moon and planets in ordered relationship within the cosmos. And a picture of our spiritual relationship with each other, and as the branches of a vine, with Christ; and through him with the Trinity. Divine ecology. All things working for good. All beautifully set out in that great ecological Psalm 104, with man in the midst.

The law of return

Beyond any conjecture, physical man is created and sustained from the dust of the earth. Then what? A few pages later in Genesis 3:19 he is informed that to dust he will return. For the intervening time, God has ordained spans of life which we now know are genetically endowed. At death the substance of all living matter will, apart from man's intervention, be broken down to become once more the dust of the soil and form the substance for new life. God is describing a cycle of life for which the laws of conservation of the land, and the return of human and animal waste exhorted in Leviticus and Deuteronomy, are seen to be crucial to health. There is great significance in the repeated undertaking by God, as the first step in the redemption of health of a people who have erred in their ways, that he would 'heal their land' (2 Chronicles 7:14). Healing commences in the living soil and is perfected in the breath of life.

A Sabbath for the land

The principle of rest from labour every seventh day is laid down and endorsed many times in Scripture. This was decreed not only for man but also for his ox, ass and other livestock. Notwithstanding the Lord's insistence on the importance of this observance, it has, down the ages, been increasingly ignored to the peril of man and his mental, physical and spiritual health.

It is fascinating to find the same principle ordained for the land, with a prescribed rest of one year in every seven. We can be sure that God would not have imposed this apparent economic hardship without a needful physical reason. We are now much better placed than were the children of Israel to understand it. We have seen through our microscopes the teeming living organisms which make up the soil. We know from analysis that the soil runs down like a battery. We can monitor how the land recovers through resting and allowing the organisms to rebuild humus and release plant nutrients.

The Lord honoured his promise to prosper his people who obeyed this Sabbath principle. He provided more than enough additional produce to make up for it in other years, and the people stayed in health along with their land. God also intended that man, by observation of nature, would learn the necessity of returning all organic waste to the land to maintain fertility. He foresaw that man would discover the advantages of composting vegetable and animal waste together before returning it to the land.

Creation—providence and precision

Central to the message of this book is the marvel of God's creation extending into the vast universe. Immediate to us is our planet, provided with an abundant supply of the materials for life in a multitude of forms, with living man at the pinnacle of this biological miracle.

It is inconceivable that having made such superb material provision God would omit to reveal to man how to live and work within the laws and forces of his creation. No manufacturer of even a modest appliance would fail to provide a handbook. But manufacturers frequently bewail that users will not be bothered to follow the instructions because they think they know it all. So it is with man in the world. He ignores, fails to see the need for, or wilfully disobeys the Maker's instructions. In his places of learning he is exhorted to accept nothing as received knowledge. He is actively encouraged to question and test everything for himself, and so he does—omitting even to accept the principles of proven and elementary hygiene, causing disease to himself and the innocent.

God's ultimate concern is for our spiritual health. But he has accorded us a temporal and physical existence on earth. His handbook for our spiritual health is the Bible. It is also the foundation to physical and mental health. Man is expected to use his mind, intelligence and powers of observation to build upon that foundation and seek out for himself the laws of the universe with the help of that most precious of gifts, the Holy Spirit, who will teach us all things needful as firmly promised by our Lord himself (John 14:26).

It is salutary to recall some of the multitude of his provisions for creation which work together to make life possible. Our planet is exactly the right diameter, and the gravitational pull is exactly right to hold on the earth's surface a mixture of gases to sustain life. Even a mile or so greater or smaller would offset this critical balance. There is just the right amount of water and water vapour to maintain an equable climate over most of the earth's surface. Air is of exactly the right constitution. (All of this and many more examples are given in the beautiful 'Fact and Faith' films.) The sun—the greater light to rule the day (Genesis 1:16)—is precisely at a critical distance to serve its purpose of heat, light and a cascade of invisible enlivening radiation. The moon—the lesser light to rule the night (Genesis 1:16)—is likewise of the precise dimension and distance to serve its essential tidal function, and it was not until man set foot on the moon that he could appreciate just what an incredibly efficient reflector this lesser light was. The surface of the moon was found to be covered in what can best be described as pulverized glass!

If the stellar and planetary system had merely happened, would it be likely that life on earth would be shielded from excessive cosmic radiation by protective ionic belts around our rolling sphere? If water was merely an unplanned product of inorganic chemistry, would it be likely to possess totally unexpected properties of latent heat, expansion and surface tension without which life would be impossible? Can we not also see the abundance of material resources on the face of the earth as predictive of man's requirements—such as atomic energy, coal, oil, wood, easily made glass and metals?

Taken with bountiful resources of food, which so readily lend themselves to intensive culture, we find the whole provision anticipates the needs of man, and is so consistently and repetitively remarkable that it is inconceivable that it could originate or continue by random chance. Yet the agnostic among us would contend that life merely adapted to what was there, and would have adapted differently had the environment been different. How little they have pondered the miracle of human life and the critically narrow physical limits necessary to sustain it. That great statistician of integrity, George Gallup, father of opinion polls, concluded that to attribute the marvel of all that makes up organic life to mere chance would be to believe in a statistical monstrosity!

Intriguingly, the Bible also describes what we have had to wait until the twentieth century to begin to unravel. The seemingly very solid objects we handle are in reality minute particles held apart by pulsating energy. Visible and tangible matter is in effect condensed energy. We read in Hebrews 11:3 that 'the worlds were framed by the word of God, so that things which are seen were not made of things which do appear'.

Life force?

I must admit to considerable sympathy with those who postulate that, among the many known forces active in the universe, there must also be a life-sustaining force of creative energy. There is considerable encouragement in such a concept from the profound statement that God 'breathed into his nostrils the breath of life; and man became a living soul' (Genesis 2:7).

We now know that everything on earth is subject to a vast spectrum of radiation with rays of wave-like motion. Only a few of these, like light, can be used by our senses. Others like infra-red, x-ray, radio and ultra-violet are detectable by instrumental means. Further extremities of wavelength and frequency are constantly being revealed. It is quite possible that we have not even penetrated beyond the fringe of knowledge concerning radiant energies in our midst.

Agnes Sanford in her book *The Healing Light* speaks of a scientist experienced in radiation who anticipates that science is poised to discover a vibration of very high intesity and extremely fine wavelength with tremendous healing power. Observing the way that God, the Master Scientist, has ordained the substance and energy of the universe, it is reasonable to conjecture, from biblical description of the breath of life and the healing forces manifest through the laying on of hands, that there exists a flow of vital and beneficial force in the creation and maintenance of life. The descriptions of the Holy Spirit in terms of tongues of cloven fire, wind and streams of living water are all consistent with a flow of creative energy. What marvels are yet to be revealed in the heavenly flow of the water of life and the tree of life with leaves for the healing of the nations (Revelation 22:1-2)?

The Almighty is seen consistently to operate within the provisions, forces and laws of the universe that he has created. He will surely not be offended if we envisage channels of prayer to and from the heavenly throne to be as real and dependable as the waves of light from the sun, the forces of gravity and magnetism.

Brian Inglis' *The Hidden Power* is further confirmation of a sense of the existence of a force, unacknowledged by conventional science, which flows through and binds together all living matter. This force he, and possibly others before him, calls 'psi'.

Divine guidance

No small part of the guidance which the Lord provides, to enable man to live in health and harmony within the system, is contained in the Old Testament law. Christians rightly accepting that they are released from the burden of the law through redemption by our Lord Jesus Christ, are in danger of making the sad mistake of ignoring the spirit and wisdom of the law, with particular reference to the extensive guidance given in the matter of health and food. Old Testament law is very much out of fashion with twentieth-century man, who dislikes the concept of original sin and tends to excuse sinful behaviour in terms of the supposed deprivations of upbringing.

Yet that law contains much precious instruction—as relevant to man's existence on earth as the law of gravity.

Guidance continues through the New Testament, revealed and interpreted by the wisdom of the Holy Spirit sufficient for all times and circumstances, 'even the hidden wisdom, which God ordained before the world unto our glory' (1 Corinthians 2:7).

Passover to health

God chose to reveal his purposes for man through his 'demonstration people' the Israelites—dealing with them by a series of covenants conditional upon faith and obedience. The march of his people through the pages of the Bible typifies—in their trials, testings and failures—the challenge and education to which we are all subject on life's pilgrimage. If the people of Israel were to survive under extremely adverse conditions, we may surely expect that God would give them divine instruction on the matter of health. This he did—early in their walk and in considerable necessary detail—as set out in Leviticus and Deuteronomy.

But so vital was the matter of health and survival that God saw it necessary to take his people in hand immediately after the passover and Red Sea deliverance. Following that miraculous crossing, God tested the people with a three-day march through the wilderness without further supply of water. When at last, parched and exhausted, they came upon water, they could not drink it! It was bitter. They rebelled in despair against Moses and God and then with death starkly facing them, God intervened again. He provided a tree which Moses cast into the water to make it sweet.

The Lord of health

And then as Israel imbibed another lesson in the matter of faith, God gave the nation one of the very first statutes, a statute of health, immediate and necessary and months before the Ten Commandments and the sanitary laws. There at

Marah (bitter), he made them a statute and an ordinance—an embodiment of the doctrine of the church and the law of the land.

> If you will diligently hearken to the voice of the Lord your God, and do that which is right in his eyes, and give head to his commandments and keep all his statutes, I will put none of the diseases upon you which I put upon the Egyptians; for I am the Lord, your healer (Exodus 15:26, RSV).

The 1949 translation of the Vulgate by Ronald Knox better reveals the preventive intent: 'I the Lord will bring thee only health.'

Thereby God is revealed in the second of his seven great Jehovah names which encompass every need of man. Jehovah-Rapha—the God that heals. The context here is undoubtedly preventive and may be regarded as God's charter for positive health.

Testament of health

The Lord follows up at once by providing two essentials of health: fresh abundant water (*elim*), and manna (I will rain bread from heaven—Exodus 16:4). Here, in addition to God's purpose of testing man's obedience, was a demonstration that food is a first requirement for health and is ideally gathered daily. Fresh food will not easily keep and, in a hot climate even kept overnight, will become putrid. What a food manna must have been, not only a wholefood but a food to provide for the body's total requirements. The promises are further expressed in Exodus 23, again conditional upon serving the Lord, that he will bless their bread and water and take sickness away from their midst. Also in Isaiah 58:11—'I will always guide you and satisfy you with good things. I will keep you strong and well' (Good News Bible).

Preventive healing

God's concept of healing is so much more than our fragmentary understanding of it. The healing of the Lord, built into every living organism, is a wonderful defensive system elaborated to protect against the multitude of assaults of a hostile environment. In terms of human health we are largely unaware of the continuing battles against invading organisms, toxic substances, radiation and adverse circumstances. Only exceptionally is conscious illness manifest. Then we may experience such symptoms as sore throat, malaise, pain, fever or rash. Even then, healing is the likely outcome. This is the healing we are aware of. The blessing of the Lord that heals is predominantly defensive and preventive and unconsciously automatic. We are no more likely to thank him for it than was the public to thank the Medical Officer of Health for freedom from the infectious diseases they never suffered. 'The Lord will take away from you all sickness' (Deuteronomy 7:15, RSV).

Compassion and healing

But the Lord is also very real in the matter of healing when the defensive mechanisms are overwhelmed by adverse circumstances. This is expressed beautifully in Psalm 103:3, 'Bless the Lord, O my soul . . . who heals all your diseases' (RSV). Our Lord Jesus Christ was moved with compassion, time and time again, when confronted with sickness, disease and disability. His instinct was to heal and make whole (see, for example, Mark 5:34).

The wisdom of the Holy Spirit

Longing to assist further, as we ponder the wisdom of the Scriptures, is the Holy Spirit who is not only able and willing to teach us but also to remind, interpret, guide, protect, vitalize and heal. Many who have sought to grapple with the wonders of the physics, chemistry and biology of the universe have been conscious of receiving enlightenment from the Holy Spirit, beyond their own understanding. Sir Isaac Newton (1642-1702) testified to receiving divine enlightenment in revealing the physical laws of gravity, momentum and

light. It appears to be the way with the Holy Spirit that just
sufficient is revealed in any generation for the requirements
and understanding of that time. The time was not ripe for
Newton to enter the realm of nuclear physics. As many
another scientist, Newton saw design: careful, methodical,
workable, elegant and beautiful design. All of this proceeding
from the counsel and dominion of a brilliant Designer. The
wisdom of health is of the Lord. 'The secret of the Lord is with
them that fear him; and he will shew them his covenant'
(Psalm 25:14).

Health, food and the law

Confidence in any book is always increased when we find it
enhances and ennobles something we already know about.
When the early chapters of such a book were written more
than 3500 years ago and confirm today's recently discovered
knowledge, that really is something! Public health, I had been
led to believe, began around the time of the appointment of
the first Medical Officer of Health in 1847. It was thrilling to
discover that public health and hygiene was expounded by
Moses (c.1500 B.C.), a great boost to my faith and trust in the
Bible as the inspired word of God. I therefore make no apol-
ogy for a simplistic approach throughout this book. As Billy
Graham puts it: 'The Bible says—and that's good enough for
me.' And the Bible indeed says in no uncertain terms: 'All
scripture is given by inspiration of God' (2 Timothy 3:16).
That clearly was also the feeling of Professor Rendle Short,
distinguished surgeon and physician, whose writings some
forty years ago I found so helpful in relating public health to
the Bible.

The way of health

The revelation of Jehovah as the Lord of health is most re-
markably manifest in the books of Exodus, Leviticus and
Deuteronomy. Here we find divine instruction, given through
Moses, for the people of Israel to walk with God in all the

ways of life, including specifically the way of health. Concerning the latter, that most spiritual of Bible commentators the Revd Dr C.I. Scofield, in his note on Leviticus 11:12, has no hesitation in saying that the dietary regulations of the covenant people must be regarded primarily as sanitary (that is, pertaining to conditions affecting health).

The instruction which the people of Israel received was far in advance of any contemporary knowledge of other nations and was instrumental in their survival in fiercely hostile conditions. It was one of the functions of this chosen race to illustrate the blessedness of serving the true God. Eventually they were to produce the Messiah to be a light to the Gentiles. Accordingly, the great divine instructions, as particularly illustrated by the Ten Commandments, have been adopted down through the ages of the Christian dispensation. With one remarkable and tragic exception: the laws relating to health and hygiene.

Three thousand years of needless tragic calamity

It is difficult to exaggerate the ravages of death, disability and disease resulting from man's continued blindness and ignorance of the elementary principles of hygiene set down clearly and precisely in the law. This whole tragic history and its consequences can be illustrated by perhaps the most remarkable of the biblical sanitary regulations, that given in Deuteronomy 23:12-14. There were to be provided designated places outside the camps for use as latrines. Every person was to carry a suitable implement to turn back the soil prior to easement, and to cover over the excrement with soil afterwards. Man now knows—as our Father has always known—that there is no more effective way of rendering excrement harmless, and free from disease-carrying flies, than by lightly covering it with soil. Very rapidly it is rendered harmless and taken back to the land as part of the humus for new plant growth and life. We often see demonstrated by man's pets the wonderful instinct of many animals to cover over their dung— even though this is sadly frustrated by our concrete jungle.

The greatest and ever present risk of undisciplined discharge of excrement and urine is the direct and indirect contamination of food and water. This pollution is essentially responsible for the spread of cholera, dysentery, enteric fever, food poisoning and many more diseases including hepatitis and poliomyelitis. It wasn't until well into the nineteenth century that any attempt was made to deal hygienically with human waste. Even in London little effort was made, as late as 1854, to prevent sewage leaking into the wells. The worst of all conditions prevailed on the battlefields; everyone has heard of the lethal squalor of the Crimean campaign and South African War. More soldiers were killed by dysentery than enemy action. Our church walls and graveyards testify to the premature demise of husbands, mothers and children, and the toll in far countries of pioneers, explorers and missionaries. The total consequences down the ages have been catastrophic. Countless thousands have died prematurely and needlessly. The confirmation of the biblical advice was not appreciated until the minute germs causing the diseases were identified under the microscope from around 1885. Even so, and through two world wars until the present day, breaches of hygiene continue to exact a heavy toll. Well into the twentieth century, horse manure falling upon cobbled streets was the direct cause of fly-borne infection of food and milk causing a grievous mortality among babies and children from dysentery.

Intriguingly, we also see the supplementary requirement to the environmental hygiene of burying the excrement, extant in Mosaic teaching—that of washing. Thousands of years before the Health Education Council, Israel was exhorted: 'Now wash your hands before you handle food.' Cleanliness was a unique pursuit among the inhabitants of the earth at that time. The synagogues were to be near a water supply. The people were to wash themselves and their clothes—there is reference to soap and lye (carbonate of soda). There was considerable emphasis on the purity of water supplies and the hygiene and covering of water vessels. Any water contaminated by a dead animal was to be discarded. Fruit and vegetables were to be washed. Man has only known about germs for 100 years. God has always known.

The Mosaic law does indeed include some remarkable wisdom relating to the prevention of infection. This is even more noteworthy since there were no hospitals, no laboratories and no skilled diagnosticians. What was required and given was a set of working rules for the priest.

There is much mention of leprosy, but this undoubtedly embraced other more infectious conditions than the leprosy we see today, which can be safely handled. Smallpox with its skin eruptions and deadly prospect would certainly have been included and would have justified the severity of the isolation. We derive the word 'quarantine' from the Levitical period of isolation: forty days. There was also the wise and essential provision for the disposal of contaminated garments now realized to be a potent source of infection.

Leviticus 15:2 prescribes as unclean, any person having a running issue out of the flesh. This would include suppurating boils, running ears, vomiting and most importantly the watery and offensive stools of diarrhoea. It would also include a main manifestation of venereal disease. Observance of the law in regard to the contained relationship, within marriage, of man and woman would be the complete answer to the prevention of venereal disease, including genital herpes with its immediate, intermittent and long-term anxiety and consequences. Furthermore, however unwelcome the pronouncement is to today's liberal generation, homosexuality was, and is, an abomination to the Lord. I stick to my contention that the Lord does not visit sickness upon sinners (or there would be none of us healthy), but an automatic penalty is liable to be exacted when there is significant departure from the ordained way for mankind. AIDS and all the fear it brings to the transgressor and the innocent is a typical case in point. The word of God is quite clear: 'Do not lie with a man as one lies with a woman, that is detestable' (Leviticus 18:22, NIV).

Why, we ask, have millions including those who knew the Scriptures down the ages failed to take the point with these diseases? Or for that matter with other lethal diseases like the Black Death which accounted for the death of millions? The clues of filth, waste and rodents as responsible are clearly given in Scripture. It certainly illustrates mankind's incredible temporal and spiritual blindness. The Lord, in both the Old and New Testament, is repeatedly saddened and angered by the moral and spiritual blindness of his people, and the trouble they heaped upon themselves in consequence.

The food laws

These Mosaic laws demand our attention no less today—though they are still hindered by blindness. They are both ceremonial and hygienic, sometimes in the same context.

Flesh

There is detailed instruction concerning meat and fish, and simple practical rules as to which species may be eaten—such as beasts which both part the hoof and chew the cud and fishes with fins and scales. Looking at some of the creatures which are thus eliminated we note this precludes the pig. There is no doubt that under primitive and desert conditions pork is hygienically hazardous as a food. Then, as now, insufficiently cooked pork can convey a dangerous worm disease, trichinosis. Furthermore, the flesh is nutritionally inferior to beef and lamb. At least one Christian author has written a book making a case against eating the pig. Likewise, and confirming the instinct of most of us, the horse was not for eating.

Shellfish are excluded by these dietary laws. I am aware that they can be very flavoursome and many people will require considerable persuasion to abstain. I have traced many cases of food poisoning to shellfish and I can also say that on every occasion I have eaten oysters I have been violently ill within forty-eight hours—not with allergy but with all the symptoms of acute food poisoning. On one of these occasions I ate oysters at a dinner attended by a large number of public health doctors. When I recovered from my illness I found that everyone who had consumed oysters had been similarly afflicted. A member of my family has also been extremely ill, suffering hallucinations akin to the described symptoms of the drug LSD, after eating crabmeat. It has gone on record in the medical press that I fear pollution of coastal waters has caused shellfish to become a very considerable public health hazard.

Looking at all the creatures excluded they tend, with notable exceptions, to be nature's scavangers, subsisting at a low level of food from waste matter.

We are certainly not justified in interpreting Peter's vision in Acts 10 as the abolishing of the dietary laws. The essential purpose of Peter's experience was to teach him that the Gentiles, hitherto regarded as unclean, must no longer be deprived of the gospel.

Fat

Of particular interest is the advice given in the ceremonial law concerning which parts of the animal may not be eaten. Much of the fat of animals is reserved for sacrifice. We can understand that the inflammable nature of fat lends itself to burnt offering, but there is good reason for believing that some fatty parts of the carcase are not good for human health, as we shall further examine in chapter 8.

Not only is the fat around the kidneys destined for burnt offering but the kidneys also, and almost certainly the liver. From a food point of view this is consistent with the biblical tendency to exclude from consumption flesh and fluids which carry waste products.

Blood

Now a word about the supreme significance of blood in the ceremony, sacrifice and atonement of our Lord Jesus Christ. Moses wrote down 3500 years ago that the life of the flesh is in the blood. The scientific truth of this God-inspired statement could not begin to be appreciated until 1628 when Harvey demonstrated the circulation of the blood whereby this life-giving fluid suffuses every tissue. Moses, having ordered that the blood was in no way to be eaten, prescribed its use upon the altar as an atonement for the soul. The significance of this will be highlighted in chapter 16 when we reach from health into the fullness of life.

It is relevant therefore to ask if there are any health reasons why blood should not be consumed—bearing in mind the repeated admonitions in the Mosaic law. Is there any non-religious justification that to this day our Jewish friends are so careful about this, with all that it involves in the kosher procedure?

The blood in its circulation is indeed the carrier of life-giving oxygen and nourishment to the millions of cells of the body. But, like the cycle of life, there is the return side. The blood carries back in the veins the breakdown products of the body which are substantially dealt with in the kidneys and liver. It can be seen, therefore, that blood in the veins is liable to contain undesirable impurities. So it makes sense that we should best avoid giving our systems the added burden of eliminating the animal's waste products. Furthermore, slaughter (however humanely undertaken) involves terror and the inevitable flooding of the bloodstream with hormones of fear which are better not consumed by man. So, although we are now, by grace, freed from any religious considerations in the consumption of blood, it behoves us to keep a watchful eye on any findings in the future which may point with more certainty to its status as a food.

The Bible abounds in reference to everyday familiar things. Most of the common foods are mentioned. This knowledge is valuable to us. We note that the blessed people of Israel manifested remarkable fitness and endurance. Their God-guided food greatly contributed to this. We can be certain that all their foods were substantially 'wholefood', and we take a closer look at them in chapter 6. Apart from modest cooking there was little or no processing. Deplete food, if any, was minimal. Yet, time and again on their way to the Promised Land flowing with milk and honey, they looked back upon and craved for the fleshpots of Egypt.

☆   ☆   ☆

. . . earth, sea and air are daily ransacked for the bill of fare.
Blood stuffed in skins is British Christians' food . . .

JOHN GAY (c. 1730).

☆   ☆   ☆

Speak to the earth and it will teach you.

Job 12:8, NIV

REFERENCE

Henry Wadsworth Longfellow, *The Fiftieth Birthday of Agassiz* (1857).

Agnes Sanford, *The Healing Light* (James Evesham 1976).

Brian Inglis, *The Hidden Power* (Cape 1986).

Rendle Short, *The Bible and Modern Medicine* (Paternoster Press 1953).

C.I. Scofield, *A.V. Reference Bible* (Genesis 2:4 note).

Doro Stell, *The Pig and You* (Jones Beeston Nottingham 1965).

6

Food for Health and Life

I now draw together my convictions concerning the essential make-up of the food best suited to the promotion of man's health in the late twentieth century. The same, in principle, as would apply in any previous century. What is not the same, and has changed more dramatically over the past 100 years than in the previous 5000, is the vast and bewildering choice available to Western man. This contrasts sharply with the frugal resources available to our ancestors, and many in the Third World today where subsistence—particularly during winter—was and is a desperate struggle.

A high proportion of the enormous amount of foodstuff now available is processed, sophisticated and damagingly deplete. Happily, having discerned, with the help of nature's open book, the essentially simple content of the body's requirements, we may hope to continue forward in the way of health, with a minimum investment of time and effort—avoiding that 'anxious thought' which the Lord expressly warns us against.

This book does not attempt to be a manual of nutrition and dietetics. It does not contain lists of food values, statistics or carlorie counts. Nutrients, including vitamins and minerals, will not be discussed in terms of source and individual requirement. Rather we shall be thinking of a pattern of eating likely to embrace all the known required nutrients and, no less importantly, those we do not yet know about, bearing always in mind the widely differing individual variations in requirement of nutrients and rate of utilization. For those who wish to have more detailed books of reference I append a couple of inexpensive suggestions at the end of the chapter.

Even orthodox nutrition has at last moved away from the static 'calorie' concept of foods. It is, however, still convenient when discussing desirable working balances to talk of protein, carbohydrate and fat. Bread—best-known of all foods which in the whole state contains so many nutrients—qualifies for a separate chapter.

Protein in perspective

This vital constituent of many foods was well named (c. 1868). The word 'protein' implies 'prime' or 'fundamental', which it is indeed for growth and repair. A recollection of school biology and domestic science, since updated by media interest, reminds us of the protein-rich foods and the discovery that some sources of protein, like fish, meat, eggs and cheese, are more complete in terms of the immediate needs of the body than vegetable sources such as cereals, legumes and nuts. This categorization into the mostly so-called 'complete' proteins elaborated in tissues of animals and, mostly incomplete, found in cereals, seeds and vegetation, has induced a much more than justifiable emphasis upon meat as an essential food.

Vegetarianism—if you so choose

I am by no means a vegetarian but do feel that we in the West overindulge in meat. Many eat meat with at least two meals a day. There are those who would feel deprived, even worried, if they did not have meat at least once a day. Vegetarians have proved the point over many generations that the best of health is attainable on a well-chosen vegetarian diet. Concern about the apparent incompleteness of vegetarian proteins is unfounded, provided variety is achieved. Non-animal proteins from different foods combine to achieve complete proteins.

High-protein diets have been advocated for a number of reasons, including weight loss. They are expensive but tend to be popular because they contain addictively tasty cooked foods. Any possible benefit to health may only be as a result of replacing the refined carbohydrate foods. We in the West are probably already eating more protein than we require. Added protein causes a significant strain in a pair of vital, heavily worked organs—the kidneys. Food surveys in the eighties suggest a move away from meat towards more vegetarianism. Many are finding that meat no more than two or three times a week is perfectly adequate. Fish is, at any time, a more than adequate substitute for meat. Other good protein meals are centred around cheese, eggs and legumes.

With the inexorable demands of the population explosion, vegetarianism is already the norm for the majority of the world's population and is likely to continue to increase in the West. It is well known that meat production as a source of protein uses many times more of the resources of precious agricultural land than does vegetable protein production.

Vegetarians argue strongly that meat eating is not healthy. They remind us of the widespread use of synthetic hormones, antibodies and tissue breakdown products. I can certainly vouch that vegetarians are far less likely to suffer the all too prevalent food poisoning.

There is certainly nothing odd about being vegetarian. When we offer hospitality we must remember that their numbers are growing and be prepared to provide for them with a minimum of embarrassment. My vegetarian friends tell me they are tired of constantly having to explain and justify their position. Many simply prefer vegetarian food without having any axe to grind. At the same time I must say that I have known vegetarians who were unenlightened in terms of the wholeness and freshness of food. They evidently assumed that the avoidance of meat was all that really mattered.

Protein: your choice

Meat, if you so desire, but in moderation. Fish, in my estimation, as often as you like. Poultry and game—as may be afforded and desired. Only very occasional indulgence in salted or smoked meat and fish. Eggs, cheese and dairy products complete the range of the familiar sources of high protein.

No less important are the wholefoods which have a valuable protein content. Milk, yoghourt, bread, cereals (not forgetting oatmeal), dried fruits, legumes and their seeds, sprouting seeds and grains.

Carbohydrate food—the well-understood misnomer

Had it not been so easy for man to extract and concentrate this energy factor present naturally in almost every food, we should never hear of the term 'carbohydrate food'. It is man who makes carbohydrate foods, not nature. Some naturally occurring foods like the cereals, the yam and the potato contain more carbohydrate than protein or fat but in their whole state do not qualify for the term 'carbohydrate food'.

Summarizing the message of previous chapters this extraction, refinement and concentration is man's single most damaging depletion of his food. With refined flour and bread there is the sad loss of a main source of other indispensable nutrients. Positively, the most damaging of all refinements is the production of sugar—white, brown or khaki—and the quantities in which it is consumed, consciously or unconsciously.

The inbuilt carbohydrate of food is intended to provide the body with a steady flow of energy without violent rises or falls of blood sugar. A heavily sugar or starch-laden meal, for which man was not designed and is not yet adapted, puts sudden strain upon the delicate mechanisms which maintain energy release and the working levels of blood sugar content.

It is not difficult, and not merely being wise after the event, to predict which organs and mechanisms are most likely to break down when civilized living has imposed more significant changes in the last hundred years than had occurred in the previous five thousand. The organ most likely to be affected by the sugar deluge is the pancreas, called upon to provide quick and sufficient releases of insulin to hold down otherwise dangerously high peaks of blood sugar. It is entirely predictable that a disease of the nature of diabetes would result and that it would have an incubation period measured in years, and affect many people. This previously rare disease is still rare in peoples where the sugar deluge has not yet arrived.

The trials to the sufferer of diabetes in day-to-day living are well known and are bad enough, but even worse is the premature degeneration which diabetes visits upon other systems, particularly the blood vessels. There is a dangerously greater liability to stroke, coronary heart disease, kidney failure, gangrene and blindness. These are some of the worst works of the 'sweet malefactor'.

Sadly, this predilection for concentrated sweetened foods affects the whole of Western society. The USA made efforts to break out of it earlier than most. I have been particularly disheartened over forty years to note the continuing blindspot of the people of Israel in regard to refinement. Disheartened because, at ground level, they are pioneers in 'getting it right' and enabling the desert to bloom and be fruitful. Yet their daily bread continues to be appalling and their feasts are filled with sugary confections. It is very difficult to obtain whole bread in Israel. They are probably spared the worst ravages of their starchy indulgence only by their simultaneous fruit eating.

Carbohydrates—our choice

The imploring message of this and earlier chapters is: enjoy your carbohydrates in a form which is as whole and naturally occurring as possible. This includes all the wholegrain products, potatoes in jacket, fruit and vegetables, dried fruit, nuts and a little honey. Be cautious and sparing with all the concentrated foods, sugars and starches (converted in the body to yet more sugar). Be wary of the many packeted breakfast cereals containing much added sugar. Reflect upon the sum total of biscuits, snack foods, cakes, pastries, puddings, sweet tea, coffee, cola and other soft drinks so customarily taken during the day. Of sugar itself, the brown varieties may have a more healthy image and may taste better but are, nevertheless, highly concentrated and to be used only sparingly.

Be kind to your children—though they may rail against you. Do not feed sugar to babies and infants. Provide acceptable fruit and vegetable 'chewy' alternatives.

Fat in the melting pot

Positive advice to the public regarding food choice, by official and semi-official bodies, is of very recent origin in the UK—scarcely more than fifteen years, with a few local exceptions. It is invariably issued tentatively, with great caution, specifies the need for further research and allows ample opportunity for backtracking.

Such food education as there is has been more centred upon fat than any other foodstuff. This is a pity, for in contrast with the simple and understandable message of the refined carbohydrate foods and the benefits of whole, fresh and raw food, the relationship of fat in the diet, to health and disease, is extremely complicated.

As we are taken through the fatty complexities of the polyunsaturated, saturated, monounsaturated, the essential fatty acids, cholesterol, triglycerides, lipoproteins, lecithin, and anti-oxidants the mind boggles at the idea of substituting highly sophisticated, factory-made oil from vegetable sources, for the milk, butter and dairy products which we were accustomed to, long before the epidemic of coronary thrombosis hit Western society and which accounts for all the frenzy about fat.

. . . as with marrow and fatness . . .

Here again, the Bible is a profitable starting point for a fuller consideration of fat. All the fat of sacrificial animals belonged to the Lord (Leviticus 3:16-17). The fat was regarded as the richest part and was rightfully appropriate for the Lord. There was also the practical consideration that the inflammable nature of fat facilitated burnt offering. Added oil is also prescribed, which assisted combustion.

Quite apart from sacrificial animals, there is a general direction (Leviticus 7:22-26) that the fat of ox, sheep or goat is not to be eaten. Distinguished physician and surgeon Rendle Short carefully considered this apparently excessive and wasteful exclusion decades before the current controversy. He reflected that the feast provided for the prodigal son included the fatted calf. Other references also suggested that cattle were fattened for festive occasions. We see that the Lord's portion of his people was: butter of kine and milk of sheep with the fat of lambs (Deuteronomy 32:14).

Dr Short then looked at the Hebrew word which described the forbidden fat, *cheleb,* which means the fat around the kidneys and abdominal organs which we call suet. This fat is very solid at human body temperature compared to the outside fat on a joint of beef or steak. We can see that it might be very wise then and now to discard this hard fat. He also observed that the pastoral Israelites consumed much fat from milk, butter, cheese and olive oil and doubtless benefited from the accompanying vitamins.

Closer to our times there is considerable evidence in the UK that the fattening of beef, sheep and pork was intensified during the eighteenth and nineteenth centuries. Massive animals were produced and every vestige of carcase, including all the fat, was consumed by a hungry population. Great heaps of suet and huge pans of rendered fat were commonplace in butchers' shops. Coronary heart disease was relatively unknown as with the primitive Eskimos who had a very high fat diet.

Today's livestock is specifically bred to carry less fat. The UK Meat and Livestock Commission to this end has instituted a pricing system which includes reference to kidney, knob and channel fat (KKCF).

The riddle of fat

Why then does it seem likely that present generations in the West are consuming more total fat than their Industrial Revolution ancestors? First, because we are mostly able to eat much more of everything than were the majority of our relatively impoverished forefathers. Secondly, because of the large quantities of 'hidden' fat taken in our convenience foods ranging across pastries, cakes, biscuits, puddings, crisps, chips, hamburgers, sausages and ice-cream.

Does it matter that fats now form so high a proportion of our diet? Studies of places like Finland where there is a high fat consumption strongly suggest an association—albeit a complex one—with the occurrence of coronary heart disease.

Are some kinds of fat thought more likely to provoke heart disease than others? This brings us right into the jungle of saturated versus unsaturated. Current suspicion is strongly directed upon the former, which include the fats associated with meat and dairy products. Why then should this arise if man has lived with these for thousands of years? It is probable that today's intensive agriculture and factory farming produces fat which is markedly different from the fat found upon our free-range ancestral herds. It is much more saturated in fact.

Should we then reject animal fat, including dairy produce, in favour of the unsaturated fats and oils available now in such profusion? First, it is necessary to be warned that by no means all the alternative fats and oils on the supermarket shelf are more unsaturated than traditional butter and cream. But even where this claim is made on the label, we have to remind ourselves of how they are made. Intensive processing is involved in extracting the oils from vegetable sources such as sunflower, sesame, safflower and corn which, in the West, have never historically formed much part of man's diet. Extraction involves repeated severe and sustained heat treatment and/or the use of solvents and various treatments to postpone rancidity. We have to remember that there are other hazards besides heart disease—cancer, for instance—connected with sophisticated food. Some of the margarines and oils carry reassuring 'polyunsaturated' labels. Others, including the first pressings of the more familiar olive oil, are described as 'cold pressed' and are less sophisticated. Even 'cold pressing' can generate temperatures higher than that of boiling water. I suspect that the ancient methods of extracting olive oil generated far less heat. We now have a whole new refinement industry extracting fat and oils from seeds such as the cottonseed which man probably seldom ate, even in the whole state.

Fat, your choice

I must say at this point that what matters at least as much as the nature and quantity of fat taken is the quality of diet in which it is eaten. I have contended for years that the worst and most damaging combination is a high-fat diet associated with much sugar and other refined carbohydrate, and a minimum of dietary fibre, fresh fruit and vegetable . . . the kind of diet very common in parts of Northern Europe, including Finland and Scotland.

My advice for most is to cut down selectively on total fat; to be particularly vigilant about the 'hidden' fats in such food as hamburgers, which are closely bound up with refined carbohydrate.

Enjoy, in moderation, the fat of butter and cream, and of pasture-reared meat. I personally do not advocate switching over to the sophisticated margarine alternatives. Enjoy some of the fat on meat, unless you are a 'Jack Spratt'. Discard the suet and dispense with most of the fat which separates on the cooking of meat. Remember always, that livestock in the wild (including fish and the fat of fish), free-range poultry and game is a splendid source of the most beneficial of all fats, the structural fats which contribute so much to the building and repair of body cells in animal and man.

Coronary heart disease is undoubtedly a matter of concern in the West. Given all its manifestations, including the furred-up arteries, the propensity to clotting and the electrical pacemaker disorders, we shall hear much more about it and about fat. It behoves us always to remember the wise, albeit chauvinistic, words of Einstein and Lord Rutherford, reinforced by Cleave, that a theory likely to be valid will be simple enough to be understood by a serving maid.

Other requirements

The foods rich in these basic components of carbohydrate, protein and fat will carry much of the body's requirements of vital substances. What of the remainder? Do we need to have a detailed knowledge of the vast array of vitamin-like substances, minerals and trace minerals to ensure we are receiving adequate amounts? Fortunately for our avoidance of anxious thought the answer is 'No'! All that is necessary is to comprehend the simple natural principles involved. To grow into a way of life where, according to opportunity and means, enjoyable wholefoods predominate in the daily choice— always including one other essential ingredient . . . the 'fresh element', as raw salad, vegetable and fruit is popularly described.

The fresh element

It has been a fascinating exercise to study healthy races, families and individuals, combining my own recorded observations with those of others, looking for common denominators, noticing how food reform appeared to be fundamental to the continued ageless beauty of so many of the Hollywood stars, and the food reformers themselves, like the radiant Barbara Cartland and Doris Grant.

I am particularly grateful for having been brought into contact early in professional life with the teachings and experience of the likes of Dr Bircher-Benner, Dr Kristine Nolfi and Dr Innes Pearse. I am now left in no doubt whatsoever that substantially raw food diets offer a significant chance of healing or partial healing in a number of otherwise intractable disease conditions. The evidence of arrest and/or regression, in a proportion of cases, of established cancer is impressive.

Understandably the raw food regime required to contend with established disease is strict and not all patients are prepared to persevere with it. Yet the beauty of identifying a routine which can heal is the potential for prevention. A much less strict regime and, for most, an enjoyable one once accustomed to it, has the potential of holding degenerative disease at bay.

The problem is in convincing people how necessary and worth while it can be to break away from the ingrained habit of predominantly cooked traditional meal patterns, especially when the rewards may not ever be fully appreciated—such as avoidance or deferment of diseases they will never know they might otherwise have got. Many conscientious mothers will require a lot of persuading that a packed wholefood lunch can be better for a child than an unenlightened hot school dinner of minced meat, gravy, tinned carrots, instant mashed potato, golden syrup suet pudding and custard—especially on a cold winter's day. Many in this generation will never be convinced.

It is necessary for education towards whole and raw food to aim for gradual change. It is better in total achievement to secure small change for the many, than dramatic change for the few. Once people have understood that cooked food should be as whole and fresh as possible; that the traditional vegetables should be conservatively cooked, then raw food can be introduced. The main course—hot or cold—lends itself to a side salad. Many restaurants now offer this—often as an optional substitute for chips or cooked vegetable. The sweet course is a recurring opportunity for such as fruit salad and yoghourt in lieu of pudding, pastry, custard and ice-cream.

How much raw food?

A realistic target for many, taking all meals into account, will be 25% uncooked fresh food. Some will soon find they can live very normal domestic, social and business lives with a 50% raw food target. The Kentons in *Raw Energy* write persuasively in favour of 75% which is equivalent to the more generous end of the diet range of the Health Farms. Although this latter regime does include many enjoyable foods—especially once the palate is adjusted—it is more likely to be adopted by those with an added incentive. Such may include those with an immediate health problem or those in stage, TV or modelling work, in the expectation that their personal appearance will be improved and sustained.

We do well to remind ourselves regularly of Dr Bircher-Benner's enduring principles: begin each meal with raw food; have some green leaves every day; use wholegrain cereals. His philosophy was that it is these seemingly unimportant eating habits, regularly repeated, which decisively influence health, not the occasional lapses.

Live food

The term 'live' is used repeatedly throughout these pages to describe food which is as close as possible to the live state in which the majority of creatures in the wild take their nutriment. In the context of man, we are talking predominantly of fruit, vegetables, nuts and herbs. When he is able to pick wild fruit, such as blackberry, or vegetable, such as tomato, watercress or radish, or herbs such as parsley or rosemary, or the ripe grains of cereals, he is obtaining 'live' food at its most fresh.

We would add for everyday purposes the whole range of fruit and vegetables, including where necessary those imported. Clearly the greater the time-lag between gathering and eating the less 'live' is the food. A few non-vegetarian foods such as carefully prepared fish may also be taken raw. Regrettably, a cautionary note has to be added in regard to the eating of raw food away from northern Europe, North America and Australasia. In many tropical and sub-tropical countries, raw food can be very unsafe unless personally prepared.

Supplements of vital substances

Where there is regular access to raw, fresh foods of these kinds, they will, subject to any soil deficiency, carry the necessary range of vital substances and minerals. This will apply to food grown on land with a good organic return and which is freshly eaten. For most of us, in town or suburbia, and especially for the elderly, there is likely to be some deficiency in our everyday eating. For this reason, I personally advocate a small range of dietary supplements: vitamin C—preferably from rose-hip and pulverized plant sources as opposed to the synthetic ascorbic acid—taken the year round and increased in winter until the spring produce comes in; wheat germ and fish liver oil, and vitamin E capsules, together with wild kelp tablets for a rich source of minerals from the sea; supplemented with the organically bound minerals zinc and selenium (since these are two minerals particularly liable to deficiency). The American super-nutritionists advocate a much longer list, including multi-vitamins.

At the conclusion of one of those all-too-rare nutrition lectures to the medical profession, the eminent bran-minded doctor who had given it was clearly rather surprised that I countenanced dietary supplements. He turned to the medical chairman with the rhetorical question: 'You don't take them do you?'

'Of course not!' was the expected response. Whereupon his young wife of fine beauty and complexion piped up: 'No, but he makes me take them!'

Dietary fibre

The same reasoning applies to the including of a sufficient amount of the now fashionable fibre in our diet. If we are on good wholefood, including uncooked vegetable and fruit, we should obtain nature's desirable content of fibre. But, realistically, since most of us consume refined and sweetened items, added dietary fibre is advisable. The most convenient form is simple miller's bran. The organic variety is preferred, thus avoiding the residues of toxic sprays which are particularly liable to lodge in the outer coats of the grain. Proprietary processed bran is unnecessary and, being usually sweetened, is undesirable. Miller's bran may be taken in milk or soup before any meal and is more palatable if some wheat germ (embryo) is mixed in with it—the latter also being valuable as a source of additional B and E vitamins. Work up from one to six teaspoonfuls daily, until you find your level.

Dietary fibre, especially in the form of bran, is the nutrition 'discovery' of the eighties. Substantial claims for its disease-preventing potential are being made. The undoubted benefits of adequate dietary fibre are: a most valuable absorbent material to assist in the necessary evacuation of human waste from the food canal, avoiding constipation; to assist in removing the toxins from the bowel contents—important in view of strong observational evidence that adequate fibre can protect against one of the most common of cancers, that of the large bowel; to contribute to the feeling of being replete after a meal, also known as satiety, and so avoiding over-consumption of refined, sugary, starchy foods. It is a sobering thought that, apart from grain surpluses, the enlightened can only buy bran and wheat germ because it has been stripped out of somebody else's food!

Stools—the unmentionable

Not a subject for undue introspection but we must be grateful to Cleave and Burkitt for reminding us that simple observation of the stools is a valuable guide to our state of health in the food canal. Where fibre is really adequate, the stools will be about the diameter of the forefinger, soft and bulky and will float in the water of the toilet. In contrast with the inoffensive stools of wildlife subsisting on natural food, the malodorous stools of man are indicative of a sophisticated, unhealthy diet—typically excess sugar in the presence of protein. Burkitt's maxim is very relevant: 'small stools—large hospitals; large stools—small hospitals.' Those unfortunate enough to be awaiting admission to hospital, especially for operation, are well advised to step up the bran intake for some days beforehand. They should insist on continuing with it while there unless, for some exceptional reason, the doctor directs to the contrary.

Where bran is taken for the first time, or the quantity is being increased, you should not be deterred by some initial flatulence—this will not last.

The Bible and the food of man

Once again I make the point that, in addition to the essential spiritual message, the Bible is a gold-mine of helpful references to assist daily living in this temporal life. It is at its richest in the matter of food: its preparation and the attitude of mind in which it should be taken. I have been much helped over the years by many of these references. More lately I have found Anne Arnott's *Fruits of the Earth* to be a delight. It also includes many recipes. We can be sure that enjoyed in moderation we are fully adapted to benefit from the foods which the Bible commends as part of the bountiful providence of the Lord, the majority of which are wholefoods.

Hallowed foods

Several foods in biblical context surely qualify to be described as 'hallowed'—none more so than fish and honey.

It falls to the beloved physician, Luke, to describe in the last chapter of his gospel the remarkable incident of the resurrected Lord requesting food shortly before his ascension. He was offered some honeycomb and broiled fish which he ate in the presence of his apostles. This was not for the purpose of suggesting that his resurrected body required material food, but a further demonstration of his bodily resurrection at which Luke, in particular, must have marvelled exceedingly.

Fish

There is abundant reference to fish as a desirable food for man and eaten with the Lord's approval. It is certainly the case that fish from unpolluted waters imparts a good measure of protective health upon people who eat it fresh and regularly. It is not only good but also delicious. It is difficult to understand how fish substituted for meat could ever come to be regarded as a fast or penance.

Honey

There is a wonderfully prophetic passage in Isaiah 7:14-15 which points to the first coming of the Lord Jesus where we are told: 'Butter and honey shall he eat, that he may know to refuse the evil, and choose the good.'

Among the fifty-eight further references to honey or honeycomb, we also note in the gospels that wild honey was a main sustenance for John the Baptist. And what more eloquent testimony to its worth than that prospect of the Promised Land to be flowing with milk and honey!

The activity of the honey-bee is one of the most illustrative witnesses to the hand of our all-loving Creator in the whole realm of the open book of nature. Beautifully expressed in words attributed to St Chrysostom: 'The bee is more honoured than other creatures not because she labours but because she labours for others.' I will always be grateful that my wife, Nancy, chose bee-keeping as a hobby during the formative years of our children. They would sit for hours near the hives watching the comings and goings, and the evictions of interlopers. They would ponder the meanings of the little dances of the incoming workers informing the outgoing of sources of nectar and other requirements of the hive. Amazingly, they were seldom—if ever—stung. In anticipation of man's need to handle the hive and the swarm, it is predictable that there would be found in nature some simple method of calming them. And so there is! Simply puffing a little smoke at them renders most colonies suitably tranquil!

Many down the ages have testified to the flavoursome, healthful and energizing properties of honey, also to its wound-healing properties now believed to be due to the enzyme inhibine. To the orthodox nutritionist, who assesses by analysing the ash left after burning, honey has little to commend itself over golden syrup, save for a few trace elements. How wrong they are! Nevertheless, although rich in health-

giving traces from living sun-drenched flowers, honey is basically a highly-concentrated carbohydrate food. If any food can
be described as homeopathic, honey is it . . . to be taken in
small quantities. Nature, by and large, sees to this. There is
only a very little honey to go round the world's vast population, unlike sugar, which can be produced ad lib. Proverbs
24:13 gets it exactly right and tells us it is good, but chapter 25,
verse 16 tells us not to eat too much of it or we will vomit and,
later, verse 27 reinforces this.

Another inbuilt miracle surely predictive of its consumption
by man is that honey, unlike golden syrup, consists of two
differing forms of sugar. The one is able to provide a quick
release of energy on absorption, the other provides a slow
release which is so helpful to the critical blood-sugar regulat-
ing mechanism—nature's natural counterpart to man's proprietary slow-release insulin which is used to make the burden
of diabetes more bearable.

For those who can afford it, honey in small quantities is a
healthy substitute for sugar. It is more whole if taken as
honeycomb, which includes the pollen complete with capping.
Many countries endeavour to avoid adulteration with sugar
syrup through legislation. There are also EEC regulations to
limit the degree of heat treatment but none, so far as I am
aware, to indicate whether or not honey has been filtered (a
process which excludes the pollen and comb solids). I must
confess, in the light of diminishing wildlife worldwide, I am
surprised at the amount of declared honey still on sale at quite
a reasonable price. Let the buyer beware!

Milk, butter, curds and cheese

All our familiar dairy products were freely used in biblical
times. Sources of milk included the goat, the sheep and the
camel, in addition to the cow. It was plentiful in the Nile delta
as well as in the Promised Land. The prime purpose of milk is,
of course, the nurture of the newborn and infant offspring.
One of its most valuable functions is in infant feeding where,
for one reason or another, breast-feeding is not undertaken or

is deficient. Milk always requires modification for infant feeding and, sadly, is liable to be loaded with added sugar for this purpose. All too often, infants find cows' milk indigestible and react with colic and vomiting. It is not surprising that allergy to cows' milk is a not-infrequent carry over from infancy. Adults, too, may find cows' milk indigestible. Goats' milk may be more readily tolerated.

Milk, being packed with nutrients, is an ideal culture and vehicle for harmful organisms. Much as I favour foods which are palatable to be taken raw, I have no doubt that the overriding consideration of hygienic safety demands that milk for public consumption must be pasteurized.

Fortunately—and predictive of man's needs, and illustrative of the purpose of benign germs as opposed to those of malign effect—there are found in nature some remarkable organisms capable of taking over fresh milk, killing off disease germs and producing valuable food with keeping properties.

Yoghourt is one of the valuable foods made possible by these so-called lacto-bacilli, cultured or self-sown and eaten by man from time immemorial. The benign germs commence the process of breaking down both the milk protein and milk sugar (lactose). Yoghourt is therefore more digestible than milk. I am happy to believe the legend of health and longevity among races where yoghourt is freely used. Yoghourt in family quantities is easily made at home. Commercial yoghourt varies greatly in sophistication and palatability. I have particularly savoured some of the yoghourts of Greece and Israel.

Another valuable product assisted by lacto-bacilli is cheese. Many a community has been helped to survive a long hard winter by cheese laid down during the spring flush of milk. But although a relatively natural food it does not suit everyone in terms of digestibility. It is also a fact that commercially produced cheese is one of the most commonly incriminated foods in otherwise unexplained headache, migraine and other allergic illness. It is, nevertheless, a tasty and nutritious food. I personally favour for day-to-day use the simple cottage and curd cheeses. In short, milk and milk products are valuable nutritious foods but, for adults, should be used sparingly.

The blessing of fruit

If there is one class of foodstuff more than any other which is generally agreed as being suitable for man, it is the juicy and pulpy fruits. By and large, doctors, dentists, dietitians, biologists, anthropologists and food reformers are now agreed that man is designed to eat fruit, that he should eat fruit and that it is good for him. It was only in the early days of dietetics and the adulation of the calorie that fruit was disparaged as being a watery mass without substance—at best only useful for thirst quenching.

The pages of the Bible leave us in no doubt as to the high value placed upon fruit, right from its first commendation to man as a main source of food in the first chapter of Genesis. God repeatedly commends the whole tree, as well as the fruit, and later provides specific instruction on the general care and nurture of fruit trees. He also urges that fruit trees must not be destroyed during operations of war—issuing the divine advice: 'For the tree of the field is man's life' (Deuteronomy 20:19). Fruits specifically mentioned include figs, dates, apples, pomegranates, olives, melons and grapes. There is also considerable symbolic reference to fruit in the teaching of spiritual truth.

The vine and the grape

Very particularly with the vine is our Lord's wonderful representation of his believers being one with him, and with each other, as the branches dependent upon the vine, and our potential for fruitfulness stimulated by the pruning of the Father. Of all the fruits, the vine and grape are a most remarkable provision of nature, responding vigorously to good conditions. The Israelites saw this during their first sortie into the Promised Land. This most refreshing and nutritious fruit would certainly be my 'desert island fruit' if I only had one choice. Short periods of relative fast, taking nothing but grapes, have been found to be beneficial to those who, by reason of travel or overindulgence, are conscious that their systems have been abused by wrong foods.

Nuts—a power pack of nature

No less worthy within the family of fruit are the nuts . . . widely used and enjoyed in biblical times, the almond being specifically mentioned. It is appreciated for the fruit, the tree and as a source of valuable oil. The roots of the trees, reaching widely and deeply into the soil, draw in a wealth of sustenance consummating in the nut as one of the richest wholefoods available to man. Mercifully also—as the squirrel well knows—they can be stored against the winter. They must be used, however, before being allowed to go rancid. They can be enjoyed in wide variety, and although they are expensive, small amounts appropriately used go a long way.

Herbs

The pages of Scripture leave us in absolutely no doubt of the importance of herbs for health and healing. There is reference to herbs in the sense of all things green, but also as herb-bearing seed. There is specific and repeated mention of at least twelve well-known herbs which have been used as food and medicine down the ages. These include onion, garlic, mint, rue, coriander, dill, mustard and balm. We also read of gardens of herbs and the desirability of having them near the house . . . which was why King Ahab said he wanted to take over Naboth's vineyard (1 Kings 21).

Many many more doubtless grew wild or were cultivated and there is proven healing virtue in herbs skilfully used over thousands of years. My appreciation of culinary and medicinal herbs is in their potential for prevention. Collectively, they make available to man a wide range of vital living substances rich in hormones, vitamins and trace elements. For those knowledgeable in their medicinal use, they are a valuable provision of Alternative Medicine. Feverfew is so highly prized as to be the object of an International Feverfew Appreciation Society. For all of us, they can be a culinary delight enhancing the enjoyment and health-giving value of raw and cooked meals. Their culinary use can also help wean the palate away from overdependence upon salt. However, they should be used sparingly (even familiar ones, like parsley) and of course when picked in the wild require accurate identification. The leaves of common comfrey, for instance, have been confused with those of the highly poisonous Foxglove.

Food reform in action

Based upon temporal and biblical observation, experience and interpretation, my plea to those not already on the road is the adoption of a measure of food reform—away from predominantly dead food towards live food. The resolve to do this may well be weakened by the 'mockers and knockers'—those who will suggest that much change will involve dull, monotonous, uninteresting, wind-filling herbage and stodge!

'How else will you endure months and months of rabbit food?' is the question posed by an advertisement for a well-known salad dressing! Nothing could be further from the truth. It has been my pleasure over the years to visit a number of proponents of whole and live foods in their homes. At their tables I have enjoyed some truly memorable meals. Delicious juices and soups, hors d'oeuvres, fresh-caught salmon trout, grilled fish of all kinds, game, free-range poultry, pasture-fed lamb, an abundance of home-grown vegetables with superb flavour, fruit salad and cream, wholemeal bread to many mouth-watering recipes, creamy salt-free butter and cheese of infinite variety, and wine (not all at one meal, I hasten to add!). And not only in private houses. What could be more tempting than this invitation to eat at a Sussex inn: 'Nothing is fried. Everything is home-made and wholemeal. Fried food is unhealthy and not traditionally English. Sauces are low in fat because we want our customers to live a long time. This is our home and people come here to enjoy our type of food, with English wine and no piped music!'

Compatible eating

For most, in my experience, the adoption of a wholefood way of life—eating in good variety according to season—is enough to provide the foundation of healthy living and a good measure of resistance to disease. For some, the combinations of the various foods taken affect their health and well-being.

One of the pioneers of food reform in the early years of this century was driven to finding his own solution through grave degenerative illness. He was an American doctor, William Howard Hay. His observations led him first—and way ahead of his time—to appreciate the importance to health of whole fresh foods. He thus secured a new lease of life for himself. But he also became convinced that it was not only the integrity of the foods which was important; the balance of foods eaten overall, and at any one meal, was also vital. The system for eating to which he gave his name and became famous was the Hay Diet. This was worked out with due regard to the composition of the natural foods available to wildlife and primitive man. A main proviso was that foods rich in starches and sugars should not be eaten at the same time as foods rich in proteins and acid fruits. To do so, he claimed, inflicted an unnatural burden on the digestive system with its alkaline juices produced to digest starch and acid juices to digest protein. Many people seem to get away with almost any combination of foods. Others, to my certain knowledge, swear to dramatic improvement from indifferent health by moving closer to nature in their food combinations.

A little before the Second World War, Dr Hay came to London in response to the considerable interest generated by articles in a national newspaper on his principle for healthy eating. Doris Grant, at his request, wrote a book of supportive menus and recipes. Lately in association with Jean Joice she has written up the essence of the Hay principles in a simple and understandable way in *Food Combining for Health*. The authors provide persuasive testimony that we would all benefit by following these essentially natural principles. Already a remarkable bestseller.

Weighing the cost

The end of a chapter praising the virtues of whole and live food is an appropriate point to mention the question of expense.

At first reckoning, the cost of such food is always greater than the commercial alternatives. Organically-grown produce may only be obtainable from the grower, and one may expect to pay at least a quarter as much more for it. Wholemeal bread continues to be dearer in the shops—but the gap is, at last, narrowing. Honey costs much more than sugar but scarcely more than jam. Taking more fruit and vegetables will significantly affect the family budget.

However, there are potential savings on the other side of the equation which can go a long way to redressing the balance. Some of us will be able to grow much of our own fruit, vegetables and herbs—and also make good use of a freezer. Some will be able to bake wholemeal bread and wholegrain cakes and puddings at a fraction of the shop prices for the less worthy alternatives. Some will make worthwhile savings on the cost of yoghourt by making it at home. And many items will progressively fade out of a wholefood way of life, with very substantial savings. These include sweets, chocolates, sugary drinks, crisps (salted potato at over £2.00 a pound!), meat paste (with dubious meat at £5.00 a pound), pastries, pies, chips, hamburgers, custard, cornflour, sauces, pickles and many more lifeless items which have no part in a healthy diet.

On top of all these savings going towards better food, we should bear in mind the immeasurable bonus of improved health for the family and the incidental savings on such as laxatives, indigestion powder, pain relievers, prescription charges, lost days at work or school and cancelled holidays.

Warranty

Subject only to consequences already incurred (personal or hereditary), I can promise any family who are prepared to reform their living habits in this way a worthwhile and recognizable bonus of health as the years go by. I have put it to the test with my own family and they in turn with theirs, and have observed the same in many others. And I by no means exclude those alone without family. I'm only sorry I cannot offer the benefit of a no-claims bonus on the National Health Service!

The Lord has created medicines out of the earth; and he that is wise will not abhor them.

Ecclesiasticus 38:4

REFERENCE

Janet Pleshette, *Health on Your Plate* (Hamlyn Paperbacks 1984).

Miriam Polunin, *The Right Way To Eat* (Dent 1978).

Rendle Short, *The Bible and Modern Medicine* (Paternoster Press 1953).

Leslie & Susannah Kenton, *Raw Energy* (Century 1985).

Denis Burkitt, *Don't Forget Fibre in Your Diet* (Martin Dunitz 1979).

Anne Arnott, *Fruits of the Earth* (Mowbrays 1979).

Doris Grant, Jean Joice, *Food Combining For Health* (Thorsons 1984).

7
Bread—the Sustenance of Life

It is a bountiful provision of nature that worldwide, and appropriate to climate and soil, edible grains can be cultivated. Wheat, rye, barley, maize, oats, millet and rice play a great part in the sustenance and health of man. This is in continuing fulfilment of the very first Bible reference to the food of man: 'Every herb bearing seed which is upon the face of all the earth' (Genesis 1:29).

Every part of these seeds, power-packed with nutrients, is valuable for health and growth. Fragmented, moistened, mixed and baked, an agreeable loaf or bread-cake can be made, which may or may not be leavened. Pulverizing the wheat may be accomplished by simply pounding with a stone or, in mass production, between millstones or steel rollers.

Bread, just as familiar in biblical times as today, was and is the hallowed object of life's greatest sermons. The bread of health is the sustenance of physical man. The Bread of Life is the sustenance of spiritual man. Bread is the divinely chosen emblem, element, allegory, analogy, simile, metaphor and parable between life temporal and life eternal.

Baker's bread, like the Christian gospel, has been continuously subject to emasculation and adulteration. Vital parts of each are sifted out in the belief that the resultant product will be more convenient to man. Bread may lose the germ, protein, vitamins, trace elements and bran; the gospel may lose the Lord's resurrection, the virgin birth and other miracles.

Our physical and spiritual health suffer accordingly.

Had this book been written even ten years ago I would have felt it necessary to devote a major part of it to continuing to make the case for wholemeal bread. The health professions sounded an uncertain note—if they thought of it at all. Indeed, as recently as 1970, a much quoted professor of nutrition was advising readers of *The Times* that the issue of brown bread versus white amounted to no more than colour prejudice. Not surprisingly, resistance from commercial interests continued. Their vast industry was geared to refining, storing and baking predominantly white flour and producing white bread and confectionery which it maintained was public preference.

The arguments over bread and flour, whole or white, in relation to health, vigour and fertility have raged from at least Roman times to this day in every country where bread is a mainstay. It has always been an emotive subject. It has long been concluded by simple reasoning that it must surely be better to retain in flour and bread the whole of the fragments of the wheat berry. Many are deeply suspicious of the motives of argument to the contrary, or scientific assurance that it does not really matter as all the nutrients are to be found in ample quantity in a 'good mixed diet'.

Until quite recent times white flour, requiring greater effort to produce, was more expensive. White bread became the prerogative of the better off, and the envy of the poor. In ignorance many were seduced down the ages from that better part of the whole grain to the impoverished status symbol of the white. A reversal of class status came in the UK round about 1870, the time of the introduction of the steel roller mills. From then on brown bread was sought mainly by those who had thought the matter through, or could afford to pay more, or who found it more satisfying.

As the twentieth century progressed, the educated and intelligent formed a fair proportion of the still small minority who chose brown bread in one form or another. It has not been until the eighties, and what might be called the 'bran bonanza', that wholemeal bread has really come into its own and has finally received official backing.

For those who are promoting health it does not really matter why people arrive at the right decisions. But it is interesting that a high proportion of those who eat wholemeal bread are likely to do so by reason of the bran cult, a slimming diet, class distinction or fashion. The fully healthful reason of securing all the wonderful richness of the wheat-berry in vital substances, minerals and trace elements is still only appreciated by a minority of a minority. The ignorant emasculation of bread has been man's greatest self-inflicted wound.

Choosing bread and flour

It is vital to health that our choice of bread should be wholemeal. This will be of 100% extraction and, when available, preferably stoneground and from organically grown wheat. Both the bread and the flour may also be called 100% wholewheat (but not wheatmeal—see below).

The disciples of the Lord, in his presence, plucked ears of corn, rubbed them in their hands and ate the seed berries— raw and uncooked. It is an educative family exercise to do likewise, after the harvest is gathered. It is delightful to chew the berries and to get the feel of their texture. A sharp knife and magnifying glass will enable the profile to be seen. Notice the soft, starchy endosperm or kernel, the little embryo or germ and the outer sac which contains them both, and is the source of miller's bran.

All parts of the berry are precious for health and the whole is a rich source of the B vitamins, vitamin E and minerals, organically bound. Stonegrinding is the method most likely to ensure all parts get into the flour. But like the famously advertised tea, once everyone gets the taste for it there won't be enough to go around! The number of stone-mills which have survived or been restored is very limited.

It is certain that there must inevitably be great quantities of flour from the roller mills to be disposed of. Much of this, as hitherto, will go to the still-large white bread market, the cake and biscuit-baking industry. Some will be sold as 'wheatmeal', a brownish meal of white flour base with a proportion of steam-treated wheat-germ put back. Some will be sold under the bran banner; white flour with added bran, in the hope that for the less well informed, health interests will be satisfied. Some such are marketed with the claim that they contain more bran than wholemeal. All these are best disregarded. As for the latter, I do advocate extra miller's bran for most of us, but do not consider bread to be the best vehicle for this.

The greater part of the wholemeal bread and flour now sold must inevitably come from the roller mills. There is returned to the end-product of white flour enough of the stripped-out wheat-germ and bran to comply with the Bread and Flour Regulations. What is unlikely to be received, and what is more fully retained in the stone-mill, is a rich and flavoursome store of minerals to be found in the crease of the wheat-berry. This is recklessly called crease-dirt in the mills and discarded. There is also the continuing liability that in a high proportion of 'shop' brown bread, the wheat-germ will have been steam heat-treated.

Manufactured wholemeal bread is of course preferable, healthwise, to white. But reluctance to make the change can be encountered, related to texture, dryness and keeping quality. I have met with this in hospitals and other institutions and have to admit that some 'shop' wholemeal bread can be disappointing, particularly when becoming a little stale.

This brings us to the controversial world of improving and emulsifying agents. Approved agents continue to be used in all manufactured bread and cereal foods, even with stone-ground flour. The most vital and precious improving agent is mercifully a natural one: yeast. The active agent of the Old Testament, leaven, which is used figuratively with pertinent effect in the New Testament. Yeast is a little miracle in itself in which God foresaw the needs of man in the making of his daily bread.

What of the chemical improvers? These have long been extensively used in the milling and baking industry. Some have been prohibited over the years. The saga of hysteria in dogs linked to agene and the dragging feet of the Ministry of Health as it was then is well known. Today's improvers are mostly on the 'E' approved list (see chapter 9). I have discussed their use with a conscientious, knowledgeable miller who provides stoneground wholemeal flour for supermarket, in-shop bakeries. The fact is that improvers are used in all the other products of the bakeries including the still-considerable quantities of white bread. He has, reluctantly, to accept that unless improvers are used in making wholemeal loaves from his flour, the public may be unwilling to buy them or come back for more. He makes the point, and I must agree, that it is far better for the public to change to wholemeal bread using improvers than to stay with white bread using improvers.

There are a few commercial bakeries who are able to produce very palatable wholemeal bread and who list on the wrapper exclusively natural ingredients, without chemical additives. One such is Goswell whose loaves are found in some Safeway Stores. Apart from these the best way to avoid the hazards of chemical additives is to bake your own wholemeal bread. For men and women this can be a deeply satisfying 'mother-earth' occupation. The resultant product is so aromatic and mouth-watering. One of my daughters, who has had to move house on numerous occasions, has discovered that one of the best ways to sell a house is to bake a batch of wholemeal bread, and when the potential buyers invariably enquire as to the aroma, offer them a taste, with country butter!

We have all heard of, and quite likely met with the veteran farmworker who points to the simple foods in his ploughman's lunch as the source of his prodigious energy into advanced old age. He refers particularly to his wife's whole bread and its staying power. He goes on to disparage 'that there factory bread' which leaves a man hungry again after an hour or so.

It is an eye-opener to visit a bread factory. Lines of white-coated operatives mixing, meting out, weighing the dough and consigning it to a large oven: and finally weighing again. How beautifully prophetic is Leviticus 26:26 to the times we live in:

> And when I have broken the staff of your bread, ten women shall
> bake your bread in one oven, and they shall deliver you your
> bread again by weight: and ye shall eat, and not be satisfied.

Bread of the Israelites

There are more than 300 biblical references to bread and it
seems that it was made daily, except upon the Sabbath. Our
Jewish friends who practise their faith continue to partake of
unleavened bread at the time of Passover. I have reflected
upon the description in Exodus 12:34 at the time of the hasty
departure of the people of Israel. They took their dough unleavened, together with their kneading troughs. Clearly at
that stage it was not only unleavened, but unbaked. We see in
verse 39 that after hundreds of thousands of them had jour-
neyed, doubtless for days, they baked their unleavened cakes
of dough. I had wondered how such a vast army could find all
the fuel and oven conditions for baking bread on the march.
Furthermore under the warm, moist conditions some of the
wheat grain would have sprouted.

I was interested recently to find in the Kentons' *Raw Energy*
a recipe for Essene Bread which enables a palatable bread to
be made through baking in the heat of the sun. The recipe
provides for the sprouting of the grain for two or three days
prior to baking. We have heard much about the Essenes since
the discovery of the Dead Sea Scrolls to add to previous ar-
chives. They were a sect living at the time of our Lord. Their
writings, from which the bread recipe appears to have been
drawn, are said to make significant reference to the healing
virtues of raw foods. Given all the occasions in biblical history
when fuel and baking facilities must have been in short supply, it is indeed intriguing to come across a means of making
an adequate and palatable bread using no more than the heat
of even winter sun in the Middle East, and which may well
have been used by the people of Israel until manna was provided. Baking in the full heat of tropical sun has of course
been known from time immemorial.

Bread: your choice

The objective to be sought is that a palatable, enjoyable wholemeal supply is available over the maximum span of a lifetime. As with other foodstuff there will be circumstances when, away from home, we have to accept alternatives. We may even choose to do so on occasion. Our reserves of health derived from a balanced mixed diet will overcome any temporary depletion. We must not worry about circumstantial imperfection. Indeed as the years go by we require less and less bread of any kind.

Nevertheless if the concept of whole bread and whole cereals has made sense with us we should lend our support to the movement away from white refined flour by requesting the 'whole' variety on all possible occasions. Millions of families and growing children will benefit once the message gets home that white bread is not the norm; people rarely prefer it once they have tasted real bread.

Bread, and the concept of wholeness it stands for, is so pivotal to health that I am here including the first and only recipe in any of my writings: the Grant Loaf. This simple and labour-saving loaf has stood the test of time. Its author Mrs Doris Grant, who ranks with the Apostles of Health in chapter 12, has done more to popularize home whole bread-making than anyone else. She was already active in this and health education during the critical years of World War Two. For those who would delve further into this fascinating subject, I list, at the end of this chapter, several of her books (together with the *Sunday Times Book of Real Bread* in which she also features).

The Grant Loaf

This recipe is based on a personal communication from Mrs Grant. There have been modifications over the years of her original recipe of which I am sure she is very tolerant. Needless to say, as with all bread, the nature, origin, hardness and freshness of the flour can account for considerable variations in the finished product. This is my wife's version of the recipe.

Imperial (metric)
3lbs (1.35kg) stoneground wholewheat flour
2 tsp or less of sea salt
2 pints (1.2 litres) water at blood heat (98.4°F/37°C)
1 tbls Barbados sugar or black treacle
1oz or large knob melted butter

Put to warm three well-greased, two-pint bread tins.

Mix the salt with the flour in a large bowl and put to warm.

Cream the yeast and sugar in a basin and add ¼ pint of the warmed water. Leave in a warm place for 10/15 mins, by which time the mixture should be frothy and singing. (If dried yeast is used place ¼ pint of the warmed water in a basin, sprinkle the dried yeast on top and leave for 5 mins. Add the sugar, mix well and leave in a warm place for 10/15 mins when it should be frothy and working.)

Make a well in the centre of the flour. Pour in the yeast mixture, the melted butter and gradually the rest of the water. Mix well—by hand is best—working from the sides until all the flour is taken up and the dough feels wet and slightly slippery. (Flour varies in the amount of water it will take up but the bread will stay fresh longer if it is rather more moist than too dry.)

When the dough is thoroughly mixed, turn it into the warmed tins. Cover with a clean cloth and put them in a warm place (not hot) to rise for 20 mins. (Warm spots can be found at the side of an Aga cooker top, a warming drawer in an electric cooker, two feet above a low gas flame or in the oven while it is heating up.) Knowing how much time to allow for the bread to rise comes with practice since every mixture varies in length of time and degrees of warmth, but as a rough guide allow the dough to rise by about one third or to about half an inch from the top of the tin.

If the bread is not allowed to rise sufficiently before baking, the loaf will be 'close'; if allowed to rise too high, the loaf will be 'spongy', could have a hole in the middle and does not keep moist so long.

Bake in a fairly hot oven (400°F/200°C) for 35-40 mins. Tapping the crust with the knuckles will produce a hollow sound when the bread is ready. Turn out from the tin on to a wire grid and leave the loaf upside down to cool quickly.

Bread for the Lord's table

God has provided man with the materials and understanding to produce the most remarkable, complete and sustaining of all foodstuff: bread. The Lord chose bread as representative of all necessary food in the prayer which bears his name. Bread has been made and eaten for thousands of years and has no rival for its undisputed title of 'the Staff of Life'—a term which derives from the Bible. It must be very significant that out of the whole vocabulary of life our Lord chose bread to illustrate his ongoing spiritual sustenance as the Bread of Life, and that he also chose bread for his divinely instituted ordinance of the breaking of bread or Holy Communion.

If it is accepted that the Lord cares, and has always cared, about the physical health of man it will not be presumptuous to suggest that whenever the food of the earth is used sacramentally to point to spiritual health, that food should be a whole and fitting element. It is thus reverently suggested that the bread provided for the Lord's table be as representative of the whole of the seed of the wheat as is reasonably obtainable.

I would not find it necessary to say more on the matter except that upon enquiry I have found that some of those to whom is delegated the privilege of securing bread for the Lord's table have not been specifically advised on the matter of choice. Others hold the belief that the 1662 Prayer Book prescribes white bread which for convenience in practice is factory-made, white and sliced.

Bread for the breaking—to whom it may concern

The compilers of the 1662 Prayer Book were wisely careful to prescribe that the bread and wine used should not be an occasion for controversy. The order for administration of the Lord's Supper or Holy Communion states:

> and to take away all occasion of dissension and superstition, which any person hath or might have concerning the Bread and the Wine, it shall suffice that the Bread be such as is usual to be eaten; but the best and purest wheat Bread that conveniently may be gotten.

I am saddened that it is the norm in so many of our churches to provide lifeless, white, sliced factory bread to represent the broken body of our Lord and sustenance of the Bread of Life. Sometimes even worse: an inert wafer of starch. Very occasionally there is to be found parochial enlightenment in this matter and a more worthy emblem of wholewheat is presented.

It is likely that the dissension and superstition which the Protestant compilers were at pains to avoid related to the issue of transubstantiation. It was unlikely to have related to the wholeness or whiteness of the flour used. There is a very great difference in the bread of 1662 and that of today. It can by no means be regarded as obligatory that 'the best and purest wheat Bread' such as was usual to be eaten in 1662 is to be construed today as the supermarket white, sliced variety. The emphasis on the definition of 'pure' in the Oxford English Dictionary is upon freedom from adulteration. This was a very considerable problem in medieval times. It is to be expected that a first concern would be to secure bread free from adulterants.

There is no doubt, by means of fine sieving, that white bread has been made for hundreds of years, but it was very much a minority bread until the eighteenth century. It also retained much more of the kernel of the wheat-germ than remains in today's white flour. In 1662 the predominant wheat bread would have been more or less brown and closer to what we now call wholemeal than to white.

White bread was one of the 'flour' prescribed grades of bread under the prevailing Assize of Bread at the time. If white had been intended there was no reason why this should not have been stated. But if white had been specified it would not be consistent with the qualifying description 'as is usual to be eaten'.

Even more certainly the bread at the Last Supper would have been a much more natural product than today's starchy imposter. The bread which our Lord broke was the Passover Loaf. Unleavened, but rich in the nutriment of the grain. (See, for example, *Last Supper* by Giovanni Salvi.)

I pray then that this and perhaps further reflection on the matter may lead those responsible for the provision of the elements of Communion to think it right to choose a loaf made from the greater part of the grain. This will be naturally brown in colour and will be better, finely milled. In the Anglican Church alone, the Alternative Service Books permit many changes from established custom. Here no guidance at all as to the nature of the bread appears to be given.

Argument, disputation or controversy would be most undesirable. Paul encountered much pointless argument over food and food customs. We can imagine he would be very scathing with this generation if we were to become similarly embroiled. God forbid that it should ever become a matter of debate by any commission or even Parochial Church Council. One can almost hear someone quite missing the point and saying: 'What possible effect on anyone's health can this tiny fragment of bread have?'

The not unworthy objective is that the bread regularly broken and shared among millions of Christians worldwide is whole and unadulterated. It must surely be at the discretion of the presiding elders or clergy so to provide. They may well choose to make the change gradually, proceeding from off-white to finely milled wholemeal.

Bread is by far our most important food.

LORD HORDER (1954).

REFERENCE

Doris Grant, *Your Bread and Your Life* (Faber 1961).

Doris Grant, *Your Daily Bread* (Faber 1944).

Doris Grant, *Your Daily Food* (Faber 1974).

Bateman and Maisner, *Sunday Times Book of Real Bread* (Rodale 1982).

Lord Horder, *Bread* (Constable 1954).

Dr Kenneth Barlow, *The Law and the Loaf* (Precision Press 1978).

Giovanni Salvi, *Last Supper* (c. 1675, Woburn Abbey).

8

Waxen Fat

Waxen fat is a rather beautiful old English description of the state of obesity. It is also found in Scripture relating to peoples who have lived and eaten well in a land of plenty, and who have forgotten the source of their blessings and turned aside from the Lord.

So very applicable to the spiritual condition of nations today, but also the serious physical problems of many of the people of the West. Waxen fat, being in a state of corpulence or obesity, is a major and distressing manifestation of Deplete Food Disease. Excess weight and unwanted flesh are most compelling motivations to an appraisal of eating habits. The connection between excess weight and faulty eating is so obvious that the slogan for the weight conscious is inverted to read: 'You are what you do not eat.'

Hazards to health

Everyone knows, especially insurance assessors, that obesity increases the risks to health. These include diabetes, high blood pressure, stroke, gall bladder disease, heart attacks, arthritis, painful joints, backache and accident proneness—although I must say that I do not wholly go along with those who maintain that our weight when we are sixty should be the same as when we are twenty.

Self-consciousness

Sufferers from obesity are all too conscious of being objects of mirth and of imputations of overindulgence. It has to be admitted that there is a lot of fatness about. The number of obese people continues to rise—at least four in every ten people in the West are significantly overweight. So much so that slimming is a multi-million dollar industry. Articles and books proliferate. Slimming clubs and weight centres abound.

Desperate measures

Cosmetic surgery for tidying up flab has been practised for years. Some, particularly in the USA, feel so defeated by obesity that they are even prepared to undergo a painful, expensive and risky operation for the removal of about nine feet of small intestine. The ghastly intent of this operation is that by eviscerating a sizeable length of gut, less consumed food will be absorbed into the system: hence further weight gain will be prevented. Hopefully there might be loss of weight. This mutilation bears the name of 'ileojejunostomy by-pass'. Needless to say the victims may find there is a price to pay for this crude interference with the anatomy of the body. Some never feel well again. This procedure is curiously similar to the mechanistic thinking behind Lane's operation of eighty years ago with the lopping out of a length of large intestine for a similarly preventable dietary condition, constipation.

Others risk taking hazardous and expensive chemical compounds which coat the lining of the intestine, thereby slowing down absorption and permitting overindulgence.

Uncomfortable facts

It is a hard fact that obesity results from taking in more food than is so required for the energy output of the body. To sufferers it seems unfair that some, who burn up energy more effectively, can apparently get away with considerable over-eating. Nor is it comforting to be told that factors like hormone balance, hereditary tendency, water balance and lack of exercise are all secondary to the necessity to restrict input in relation to our own personal output until we get near to a normal weight for our height, and stay with it.

Unhealthy associates—starch, sugar and fat

There is a category of food which, more than any other, is responsible for a great part of unwelcome obesity. I refer to the refined carbohydrates which include sugar, sweets, confectionery, syrup, jam, white bread, white flour, polished rice, sago and tapioca. These are worst of all when combined with fat as in biscuits, pastries, puddings, fried bread, hamburgers, chips, cream cakes and ice-cream.

And you shall eat and not be satisfied (Leviticus 26:26)

Whatever interpretation may be put upon the verse from which these prophetic words are taken they are very fitting to Western man's position today in relation to his excessively refined food. It lacks bulk and fails to communicate to the stomach that feeling of repleteness which comes from food with a natural proportion of fibre.

The old English word 'satiety' exactly describes what occurs following a wholefood meal. With refined food, before any feeling of adequacy is felt, the chances are that an excessive amount of fattening calories will have been consumed. And because it is refined it is absorbed quicker than nature intended and a feeling of spurious hunger is experienced much too soon again. The food lacks staying power. This can account for much of the compulsive eating of which an obese person is only too aware.

The refined carbohydrate foods and their fatty partners are deceivers of tongue and appetite. Sugar is the most empty of all the available calories, the degree of refinement being some eight times greater than in the case of even white flour.

Sugar alone is more than sufficient to account for much of the obvious obesity seen. In Britain we consume two-and-a-half million tons of the stuff each year. We take it not only as the sugar we can see but in every conceivable hidden form in convenience foods, confectionery and soft drinks. It is taken in considerable quantities as malt sugar in fermented liquors such as beer. More than 2000 pints are consumed each week in the House of Commons alone, a place well known for over-eating. A sabotage scare revealed the astonishing fact that three million Mars Bars are eaten daily in the UK. We also average nearly one-and-a-half gallons of sugared and fatted ice-cream per head each year. The Americans consume an even more incredible five gallons per head.

In the wild, except for very limited and guarded supplies of wild honey, nature only permits the animal and bird kingdom to savour sugar when bound up with a considerable quantity of pulp, fibre and roughage as in fruits, sugar canes and root beets. Man alone can extract it. No animal can obtain refined sugar unless given it by man—as he delights to do to his pets, horses and zoological captive animals.

To obtain his daily average of six ounces of sugar, man will have discarded some three pounds of fibre and roughage. Not that the roughage of the sugar cane or sugar beet cropped specifically for its sugar content can be made palatable for eating, like miller's bran. But it is to be noted that native communities who chew sugar cane do not succumb to such Western scourges as diabetes and dental disease unless they also consume Western refined foods.

Fattening hospitality

Sweetened drinks, cakes and biscuits are a common form of inexpensive hospitality in the West. They are proffered daily in the home, at social events, in parish halls, garden parties, workplaces and business houses. These comestibles are al-most invariably refined and sweet. An occasional indulgence for the sake of fellowship or courtesy may be all very well, but for those regularly involved in house calls, social events and the like, the result can be devastating to the figure and to health. Refusal of the hospitality offered is liable to give offence and may certainly be counter-productive in other respects if the visit is one of friendship or compassion.

I have before me a recent press cutting carrying a photograph of a large and ample clergyman. The story of his addiction to sweet offerings was picked up from a church magazine. This contained a heartfelt message from his wife to the parishioners, informing them of his sweet tooth and rising obesity, and pleading with them to refrain from leading him into temptation!

The message for all of us is that we reform our traditional but bad food habits, and offer a minimally sweetened wholegrain biscuit or the like by way of hospitality and example.

I can anticipate impatience and resentment that I am daring to point a finger to such commonplace and seemingly harmless customs in the Western way of life. I am almost certain to be regaled with more stories of inveterate cake and biscuit eaters who broke all the rules for a lifetime and who survived to ninety-five—hale, slight and hearty—with all teeth intact! I do not retract. The quantity of refined, deplete food eaten at elevenses and minor social occasions between meals is prodigious and, when continued year after year, must contribute to Deplete Food Disease of which obesity is but one manifestation. The old English proverb is very true: 'Often and little eating makes a man fat.'

The villain—but not the only one

The refined carbohydrates are thus seen to be at the heart of most obesity because of their artificial concentration, cheap availability and the addictive taste which is inherent in the sweet malefactor. At the same time it must be stated that there were fat people around long before the commercial refining of carbohydrates. Shakespeare saw and portrayed them in words, as did many an artist on canvas. Eglon, King of Moab, is described as a very fat man in the third chapter of Judges—so much so that the fat of his belly closed over the haft of the sword which killed him and could not be removed by his assailant. Obesity of long ago was confined to a small minority having the wealth or opportunity to indulge in gluttony.

Likewise today, all or any food overindulged can lead to obesity. Fat and oil remain important contributors to corpulence. Fat lends itself to refinement and extraction. An elementary and time-honoured process of the separating off of fat is to remove the top of the milk for processing into cream and butter. Fat is a product of cooking meat. Housewives have a compulsion to re-use it. Most of it would be better discarded. Animals in the wild have little opportunity to indulge in fat.

Man also extracts numerous fats from seeds and grains— some of which, like the oils of groundnut, corn, safflower, grapeseed, fish and cottonseed, are only a recent source of food for him. Some of these are processed into margarine and cooking fats, extensively used in the home and in commercial foods. By and large, fat is more than twice as weight-promoting as either carbohydrate or protein.

The protein foods are delectable to man. Many in the prosperous West consume considerably more protein in the form of steaks, hamburgers, joints of meat, poultry, bacon, eggs, fish and cheese than the body requires. A high-protein diet will only assist weight control if the protein replaces carbohydrate and fat which would otherwise be taken. It is not particularly to be commended and does not represent the basic food for which man was designed.

Calories—easy to come by, hard to lose

Numerous publications go into considerate details regarding the calories contained in the various foods and their respective fattening or slimming potential. Calorie counting is a time consuming and boring business and many give up and lose count, and heart. Nevertheless for those with a serious problem of overweight a food value fact book will be an advantage. One such readily understandable book which can be helpful is *F-Plan Diet*. F stands for fibre which is presented as a late twentieth-century discovery of medical science— whereas, as we have seen, God built necessary fibre into food from the beginning. Foolish man extracted too much. Wise observers have sought to restore it over at least 150 years.

Scales, both bathroom and kitchen, occasionally used, are also useful but food intake is not meant to be an exact science. What is required for most of us is a day-to-day, rule-of-thumb, working knowledge of the good and whole foods in moderation. Remember that when an extra large appetite calls, whole and raw fruits, salads and vegetables provide satiety, are not fattening and are the bearers of the best components of living food.

There is an obvious relationship between weight control and physical activity. Yet most people are aware and rather depressed by the fact that an uncomfortable amount of exercise is required even to burn off the calories of a few extra lumps of sugar. The fuller implications of exercise are dealt with in chapter 10.

There is also a general awareness of psychological and familial factors in the matter of obesity. Some are a hangover from infancy. Mothers mistakenly equate plumpness with health and instil feeding habits accordingly—including the sweet tooth, initiated by that appalling practice of lacing cows' milk with sugar for bottle-fed babies. (Proprietary feeds modified with lactose are preferable.)

For others, food—especially the kind once lavished by mother—is a symbol of love and affection. Overindulgence continues as we reward ourselves when human love is scarce. For some such, the realization that Jesus can provide the love being sought can be a turning point.

At least one evangelical movement in the USA has considered the frustration and despair of many of the seriously overweight who fail in their own strength, time and time again. Sufferers are encouraged by the fact that the Lord is concerned over personal health and the maintenance in this earthly state of a fit habitation for the Holy Spirit. Those who successfully place this burden with the Lord rejoice in the company of 'Overeaters Victorious'.

☆   ☆   ☆

Whatever may be the quantity that a man eats it is plain that if he is too fat, he has eaten more than he should have done.
DR SAMUEL JOHNSON (c. 1775).

REFERENCE

Audrey Eyton, *The F-Plan Diet, Calories and Fibre Charts* (Octopus Books/Marks and Spencer 1983).
Marie Chapian, Neva Coyle, *Free to Be Slim* (Kingsway Publications 1985).

9
Additives, Allergies and Addictions

Attention has so far mostly been directed to the missing substances in food as a cause of disease. Turning now to the other side of the coin it will come as no surprise to be reminded that additives in food, taken consciously or unconsciously, can be a very real menace.

Contaminants

These are incidental additives which are picked up by food mainly in the growing and storage processes. They arise from a world use of organic chemicals amounting to millions of tons each year for the control of insects, rodents, fungi and the whole range of plant and animal diseases. They include pesticides, antibiotics, growth-promoting hormones and biocides. Some, such as the organochlorine and organophosphorus pesticides, are powerful and persistent.

Given the world as it is, rather than how we might wish it to be, and given the enormous population concentration to be fed, we can take it that most commercial food is subject to a considerable and increasing number of such contaminants. No small effort, nationally and internationally, will continue to be made to monitor adverse effects of these upon health, but inevitably some will be more susceptible than others. This subject will not be pursued at length lest that very anxiety and concern be fostered which it is a main objective of this book to minimize.

Additives

A vast number of chemical substances are purposefully added to food. Nearly all items of a convenience nature or requiring a shelf-life will contain some. So much so that it is estimated that an adult will unwittingly consume on average eleven pounds of additives each year. We are reminded of them whenever we see the code letter E on a food package. E stands for many things but in this context we might think of explosion, equivocal and extraneous, as we consider the ever-increasing number of additives and the dubious and uncertain consequences of many of them.

E for extraneous extras

> INGREDIENTS: Sugar, Tomato Powder, Modified Starch, Dried Glucose Syrup, Salt, Vegetable Fat, Dried Milk Powder, Flavour Enhancer: Monosodium Glutamate, 621, Caseinate, Acidity Regulator: E340, Emulsifiers: E471, E472(b), Colours: E124, E102, Malic Acid, Antioxident: E320.

We remind ourselves again at this point that we are seeking the simplest possible way through the food jungle, compatible with health. We are endeavouring to avoid undue worry and concern about our daily food. Even so, we will be fortunate in our choice of available food if we are not from time to time confronted with a label like this, typical of thousands on packages on the supermarket shelves. Additives have been proliferating for years. These include some hundreds of colourings, preservatives, antioxidants, emulsifiers, stabilizers and flavour enhancers. Their main purpose is to enable food to be preserved and readily saleable without liability to the growth of harmful organisms or moulds, also to render food attractive to the eye and of good consistency. Less worthy use is the chemical substitution of natural ingredients with flavoured artificial substitutes or the adulteration of such as ham and poultry to cause it to hold more water.

The particular label extract above is taken from a sachet of instant cup soup dominated by an appetizing tomato-coloured picture. Not much in the way of healthful nourishment we might conclude, and what are we to make of the letters and numbers?

Increasingly (and much overdue) food manufacturers are required to disclose on the package the ingredients of processed food. Numbers are being allocated to these hundreds of additives, to make it possible for the consumer to exercise some discrimination. To assist understanding of the code, there are now several publications which indicate the not inconsiderable number of those liable to be suspect, the equivocal ones, and those likely to be safer. The latter will include colourings such as: chlorophyll, E140; Iron oxide, E172 and Vitamin B2; E101 (tartrazine); E110 (sunset yellow); together with preservatives like acetic acid, Vitamin E, E306, Alginates from Seaweed and Pectin E440. Increasingly, the numbers quoted will bear the prefix E denoting their permitted use throughout the EEC.

The best possible way to avoid worry and concern about food additives is to make up the main meals from freshly-produced food. Best of all, from genuine organic suppliers. This may include fresh fish (as opposed to dyed, smoked, salted kippers). Mercifully the 'goodwill of health' established by such food, including the raw fresh element, will fortify the natural defences sufficiently for most of us to accept hospitality without embarrassment and of necessity partake occasionally of convenience foods.

Indeed it seems that a majority of consumers can live with additives and contaminants for years without conscious or recognizable consequences. A minority may be allergic or sensitive to them (which we will look at shortly).

Salt—a major risk factor

Salt is the world's most common and extensively used additive. We are reluctant and remarkably slow to accept the mounting evidence that an excess of what is an everyday and seemingly innocent white substance, freely used in our kitchens and at our tables, may be responsible for a great volume of premature disabling diseases and deaths. Most of us ingest very considerable quantities of salt in foods already prepared and the practice of shovelling even more salt on to food is commonplace. Addiction to salt is widespread. Including all the salt added for preservation, manufacture, cooking and taken at the table, modern man consumes at least five times as much salt as is good for him.

Ancient man also had a partiality for salt. More than four thousand years ago Chinese physicians observed that if too much salt is used in the food the pulse hardens. This points to the consequence of raised blood pressure and greater liability to premature degenerative disease such as a stroke.

Racial studies worldwide strongly suggest that peoples who traditionally use much less salt maintain low blood pressure throughout life. All races who overindulge in salt are prone to a rise of pressure with age and greater liability to stroke. It is not really surprising that the body's delicate tissue balances should be upset by excess salt, thinking back to school science and the powerful osmotic effects of salt solutions.

Reduction in salt intake can produce a marked fall in blood pressure for some people. In others, the blood pressure threshold remains raised. This alternative response is probably of genetic origin but the difference has delayed the advancement of a consensus view among the health professions who were looking for a simple cause-and-effect relationship.

I have no hesitation in urging that most of us should cut down considerably on this self-chosen additive. Including sophisticated foods and cooking, many are consuming at least five teaspoonfuls of salt each day. We should aim at no more than one teaspoonful and start by not adding salt at the table. A greater use of herbs and spices in cooking will enable substantial reduction together with the avoidance of snacks such as salted nuts and crisps. Above all it is important to use fresh whole foods, and the enjoyment of natural flavours will develop as the palate recovers from years of salt addiction. To assist in the necessary change of habit, potassium-based salt substitutes are permissible.

Allergy and addiction

Allergy and sensitivity to foods such as strawberries and shellfish have been recognized for many years. Reaction to pollen and housedust and the familiar manifestations of hay fever, eczema and asthma are all too familiar.

Less well recognized is an epidemic of sensitivity and reaction to chemical agents in food and in the environment. Failure to recognize this partly results from a much less obvious cause-and-effect relationship. Addiction to some of the agents and apparent relief of symptoms with renewed dosage is at last being recognized as masked allergy. As with all new findings, considerable controversy rages as to the extent and reality of these manifestations. The number of doctors experienced in the new discipline of recognition known as clinical ecology is very limited. What is certain is that there has been in very recent years a dramatic increase in the number of chemical stimulants with which we have to cope, including the food additives.

When we are feeling less than well there is a tendency towards hypochondriasis in all of us. It is tempting to say: 'Of course! That's it! No wonder they can't account for my symptoms. I've got a food allergy and they don't even recognize it.'

I must not do more than suggest that where recurrent symptoms of a transient and bizarre nature are experienced— for which on investigation no organic cause has been established—then the possibility of food or chemical allergy should be borne in mind. Even to indicate the nature of the symptoms can be misleading, but in the most general terms they might include swelling of varying parts of the body, unaccountable sweating, racing pulse, migraine, wheezing, sensations of panic and tension.

Where there is good reason to pursue the subject further, I recommend two paperbacks by Dr Richard Mackarness, a perceptive psychiatrist who concluded that the cause of the symptoms of many patients referred to him was by no means all in the mind.

Under medical guidance a main plank in diagnosis and

treatment is a process of elimination. Patients are put on a basic Stone-Age diet starting with spring water and a period of fast. If symptoms disappear it can be suggestive of the implication of one or more foods. Items are then restored to the diet one by one, noting if symptoms reappear. Apart from the successive exclusion by trial of a few of the well-known allergens such as coffee with its caffeine content, tea with its caffeine and tannin, chocolate, eggs, cheese, cows' milk and products, and wheat products, these elimination diets are not really suitably conducted on a 'do-it-yourself basis'.

I would accept that some foodstuff taken in the most natural of states can give rise to sensitivity. I strongly suspect, however, that for the greater part this increasingly recognized epidemic stems from deficiencies in the body's immune systems due to missing building-blocks in the food supply or from contaminants, additives or sophistication of the offending food items. In short the better the integrity of your whole, live food intake the better chance you have of avoiding allergies.

Drugs

What a multitude of substances are covered by this emotive word. They are certainly additives to what is normally taken into the body. We can become addicted to them and they can be responsible for allergic reactions.

I leave it to others to answer the question as to why the world is in the grip of a terrifying epidemic of the taking of hard, mind-bending, lethally addictive drugs, particularly involving young people. I suspect, however, that some of the blame can be laid at the door of deficiencies in the daily food.

There is a prevailing epidemic of dependency upon tranquillizers, sleeping pills, antidepressants and stimulants. Millions upon millions of prescriptions for these are issued each year and millions more for other remedies. Additionaal remedies bought over the counter add up to a dismal picture of a tense, stress-laden, allergic, catarrhal, indigestive, constipated, sleepless community. Turning out the medicine cabinets of deceased persons is quite an eye-opener.

All of which is very sad, because the fact is that, apart from the use of a very few drugs specifically and usually for short periods, the taking of medicaments has no part in health care and if simple healthy ways of living are followed they are quite unnecessary. I have observed this over and over again in healthful families. I have also observed that the taking of drugs for temporary symptomatic relief can be a cause of illness, especially when several are taken, perhaps unknown to the doctor, and they react together. A doctor friend of mine finds himself constantly astonished at the number of drugs patients are taking when they arrive in hospital. Invariably his first act is to take them off all drugs and some are very much better in advance of any other treatment. Being made ill by the supposed cure is sufficiently common for there to be a word for it in the medical dictionaries: 'iatrogenic'.

There are some very well understood reasons why drugs can be debilitating. They are all toxic to a degree. Many make heavy demands on the body's resources of nutrients—especially the vitamins and trace elements. Drugs, specifically sedatives, tranquillizers and antihistamines, can have a marked effect upon performance, being especially hazardous as a contributory cause of road, industrial and home accidents. Alcohol is rightly monitored in relation to driving. It is no less important that measures be put in hand to discourage from driving those under the influence of drugs—whether for theraputic reasons or otherwise.

The contraceptive pill

It is not within the scope of this book to advise on the acceptability or otherwise of the contraceptive pill. I confine observation to suggesting that where it is taken some of the side-effects may be less troublesome or threatening if the daily food is of the whole and fresh variety advocated in these pages, taken together with some additional miller's bran. It is possible that the slightly greater liability to clotting within the blood vessels may thus be diminished. The avoidance of smoking is of course no less important.

Alcoholic drinks

These qualify for inclusion under all three headings of this chapter. Alcohol derives from the natural process of fermentation which is widespread throughout nature and is part and parcel of the breakdown process of organic material in the cycle of life. Fermentation at its most basic level is what lends the heat to our pile of mown grass. It is certain that man and animal have adapted over thousands of years to alcoholic fermentation.

Wine and beer

Wine is derived from the controlled fermentation of fruit, herb or vegetable. Fermentation of grape juice produces the most palatable and most widely consumed of the resulting wines. Enormous quantities of grapes are grown worldwide specifically for wine-making.

Wine was a widely used commodity in biblical times and apart from specific occasions such as for the priests before the altar there was no prohibition of its use. Indeed the prohibition of wine with its built-in resistance to the carrying of disease-causing germs would have been a harsh and impractical requirement under conditions where there was so little pure water available. Wine is commended in moderate use as a gift from God to gladden the heart of man. But there is repeated warning against excessive indulgence and drunkenness. And we see how the very elect of God can be overtaken, as with a drunken Noah in the first Bible reference to wine in Genesis 9.

Then, as now, true temperance in the matter of wine is moderation and, taken accordingly, good wine can enhance the enjoyment of food and enable us when meeting socially to get on better with fellow human beings. There are claims that wine can reduce the liability to coronary heart conditions. If this is so, one probable reason is that wine provides traces of nutrients which are otherwise deficient in civilized living—chromium for instance.

For those of other tastes the fermented malt liquors providing barley wine and beer are alternative beverages where the strength of alcohol is also restricted by the limits of the fermentation process. The alcoholic content of wine averages about 12% and beer and lager about 4%.

Spirits

We move into another dimension in the matter of alcohol when we consider the spirits. These are made by distilling fermented liquors to produce drinks of a much higher alcoholic content. Wine distilled in this way produces the brandy family. Distilled malted liquor produces whisky, while fermented grain or vegetable matter distils as gin. Fermented sugar-cane products come over as rum. The alcoholic content of all these as sold averages about 40%. In between wines and spirits are the fortified wines like sherry and port. Spirits are used in their preparation to lift the alcoholic content to about 20% by volume.

The other side of the coin in regard to health is the undeniable fact that, for a minority, alcohol is liable to become an addiction, and taken in excess it will have serious consequences in personal and family life. There can be a grave risk of violence and injury. There are almost always psychological factors involved.

My considered opinion in the matter of alcoholic beverages is that as man's body is conditioned and has been adapted over thousands of years to basically fermented wines and beers, moderate indulgence is for the majority unlikely to give rise to health problems. For those who succumb to prolonged abuse, one of the serious risks is damage to the liver. Women have the greater liability—possibly because of a smaller physique.

Distilled spirits were not mentioned in biblical times. Man's time for adaption to them is measured in hundreds of years at the most. Habitual drinkers not uncommonly take spirits neat although some dilution is more usual. Either way the likely alcohol level is liable to be damaging to the delicate membranes of the gullet and stomach. There is also a greater liability with stronger drinks to consume more of the toxic by-products of fermentation and distillation, which can be more upsetting to some than the alcohol content. In short, those who wish to minimize the stresses upon their tissues do well to be careful in the use of spirits.

Perhaps the most valuable use of spirits is as a late night-cap for the elderly to assist sleep without resorting to drugs.

The only other point I would make is that beer and some wines are rich in carbohydrate and can be considerably fattening, and that all alcohol should be avoided during pregnancy, breast-feeding and when performing skills upon which the lives of others depend—such as driving and flying.

Finally, to mention again in the particular context of alcoholic drinks, the importance of avoiding disputation among Christians. Total abstinence can be an occasion for witness but over-virtuously presented it can have the opposite effect. As in the matter of food and circumcision Paul was greatly saddened by unnecessary controversy. We ought not to be divided as to whether or not wine may be taken, when God's only direction is that we avoid excess.

☆   ☆   ☆

Leave thy drugs in the chemist's pot if thou canst not heal the patient through his food.

HIPPOCRATES (c. 360 B.C.).

REFERENCE

'Look Again at the Label' (Special Report by the Soil Association 1984).

Richard Mackarness, *Not All in the Mind* (Pan 1976).

Richard Mackarness, *Chemical Victims* (Pan 1980).

Maurice Hannsen, *E for Additives* (Thorsons 1984).

10

The Breath of Life and the Profit of Exercise

Having insisted that over the span of life we are what we eat, it is necessary now to remind ourselves that the body's most immediate and continual contact with surrounding nature is with the air. We can survive, if need be, without food for several weeks, without water for several days, but if we cease to breathe air for only a few minutes irreversible changes occur in the system followed usually at once by death.

Most people when asked the purpose of breathing will say that it is to get oxygen into the blood via the lungs. This is correct in so far as it goes, but most, when asked what propels the blood via the arteries to the tissues and back via the veins, will reply to the effect that it is the heart's pumping action. But these conceptions only include half of the essential requirements of breathing and the circulation of the blood.

We all tend to overlook that the main purpose of the heart-pump is to push the blood outwards right to the uttermost tiny hair-like capillaries. Its pressure is finally expended in the tissues; the heart can have very little to do with getting it back again. No, it is the action of the body muscles pressing upon the veins, which have one-way traffic valves along their lengths. This action serves to push the blood back towards the heart-pump supplemented massively in the last lap (as the returning blood reaches the abdominal cavity) by the action of that seldom seen muscular sheet, the diaphragm, which separates this cavity from the lung cavity.

This muscle, acting in conjunction with the muscles of the rib cage, constitutes the vital breathing pump. When we inhale, the diaphragm descends like a piston and raises the pressure in the abdomen forcing the pooled blood in the huge veins up into the heart chambers, assisted by the then expanded chest cavity.

The purpose of this little homily is to remind ourselves of the absolutely crucial part played by the breathing process upon our daily health. Not only to oxygenate the next round of blood as it is pumped through the lungs, but to play the dominant part in getting the used blood back to the heart and lungs. Impaired mechanical circulation of the blood is more often due to faulty habits of breathing than to any deficiency of the heart. Shallow-breathing habits (apart from repose and sleep), and also breath-holding, are significant causes of preventable strain upon the heart.

Breathing is a bodily function which we are able to control both voluntarily and involuntarily. Today's all-too-prevalent minor stresses can result in breath-holding and can also have the opposite effect of encouraging rapid breathing from the upper chest and some quite curious symptoms caused by over-breathing.

Both of these breathing habits are bad for those whose physical activity is largely confined to the office, factory, car or home. We all need to cultivate a relaxed slower breathing pattern involving the lower chest, diaphragm and abdomen with an ample full expansion and contraction so that the breathing pump can perform to the full its job of helping the returning blood. The movements of the chest wall and abdomen can be monitored with the palms of the hands—sliding them down on to the abdomen during expiration and assisting the drawing-in process and feeling the abdomen expand as full deep inspirations are made.

The proper working of the abdominal breathing pump is especially important where there has been damage to the heart from coronary thrombosis or any other cause. But best of all, it helps to prevent damage in the first place.

The exercise myth

The cult of exercise and physical fitness continued to be an uppermost thought in the minds of the Greeks at the time of Paul's travels. Some of their fine arenas and running tracks had been established centuries before his time.

It is inevitable that he would consider the relevance of exercise to man. He puts it firmly into perspective:

> Train yourself in godliness; for while bodily training is of some value, godliness is of value in every way, as it holds promise for the present life and also for the life to come (1 Timothy 4:8, RSV).

The Authorized version is even more dismissive of exercise: 'For bodily exercise profiteth little.' Earlier in the same chapter Paul points to a time to come, which could well be here and now, when there will be a departing from the true faith in favour of diversionary cults. Certainly in the West we are back to the cult of the marathon to which we add the work out, frenzied dancing, jogging, aerobics and the 'exercise burn'. There seems almost to be a pursuit of elusive joy in physical stress and pain.

We note Paul's other observations of the marathon and the games. The exercise of strict control by the athletes to receive a perishable crown. How much better to receive the imperishable crown of life (1 Corinthians 9:24-25).

Today's craze for exercise to the limit has probably been encouraged by several controlled trials which suggest that the liability to succumb or die from the prevailing epidemic of coronary heart disease is lessened where exercise is a part of life as opposed to the sedentary existence.

It is well established in nature that parts of an organism which are not used tend to waste away. It is desirable that we regularly use as many of our body muscles as possible. Many observers have testified that daily walking is one of the most effective means of achieving this. Walking is recognized as a valuable means of rehabilitation after a coronary attack and I am convinced that no small part of this benefit derives from the exercising of the breathing pump. But I do not find convincing the extrapolation that because moderate regular exercise is good for physical health, vigorous burning exercise to the limit of endurance must be even better.

The hazard of irregular exercise

Indeed I hold a directly contrary view. Strenuous exercise, especially if only spasmodic, can be lethally dangerous. Those of riper years sometimes talk of their regular exercise. On questioning, 'regular' turns out to be once a week. Exercise, to qualify as regular, needs to be almost daily, and one needs to work up to this. Weekly work-outs of squash, tennis or even golf can be hazardous. There is no evidence to suggest that strenuous exercise promotes longevity. On the whole, world-beating athletes do not achieve anything like the longevity attained by orchestral conductors whose chest muscles are so beautifully exercised. I do not mention this in order to deter young people from exercise. Indeed I have for years railed against the growing practice of children being driven around unnecessarily in cars by overstressed parents.

I do contend, however, that exercise to the limit on the endowment of a poor diet can be dangerous. It can happen to racehorses too, apparently at the peak of condition, and surprisingly even to horse riders under exertion. A classic recent example relates to a young woman show-jumper who collapsed and died in action. The post-mortem showed little or nothing and for want of a firmer conclusion, a diagnosis of 'spontaneous cardiac arrythmia' was made. The pathologist is reported to have stated that we will probably never know exactly what caused it. He concluded that it is one of those things which happen from time to time in completely fit and healthy young people!

But are such casualties really completely fit and healthy? My observation is that disturbed rhythm of the heart, long-term or sudden, can be predicted simply through a deficiency of some vital ion required for the full functioning of the heart's electrical system. A likely manifestation of a greater or lesser degree of Deplete Food Disease.

That most perceptive family doctor, Walter Yellowlees (see chapter 12) in his brilliant 1978 Mackenzie lecture also puts occupational exercise in perspective. He has been appalled, over the years, at the exceptionally frequent occurrence of, among other degenerative conditions, coronary heart disease in the lovely rural Highland Valley of his practice in Scotland. He notes that farmers and farm workers are no more immune than others. Their active outdoor work seems to afford them no significant protection against living in one of the worst risk areas for coronary heart disease in Europe.

Yellowlees has no doubt that the biggest factor is the Highlander's appalling diet. Theirs is a massive addiction to the refined carbohydrates. He is amazed that farmers, who devote so much effort to providing the best food to produce salable and prize-winning farm animals, encourage their wives to load their table with devitalized factory food oozing with fat, sugar and starch.

Coming back to walking, this is an opportunity either for solitary contemplation or for uninterrupted human companionship. Also man's closest animal friend, the dog, can most effectively encourage him in this exercise.

In passing I must add that there could scarcely be a more perfect illustration of the kind of devotion, loyalty and obedience which man owes to God than that which man can receive from his dog. Furthermore, it comes as no surprise that the surely divine ability of a wide variety of animals, especially the dog, to become the pets of man, is seen to be of benefit to human health. Their ability to supplement human companionship is a gift of God. The stroking and fondling of animals is recognized to be of benefit to health. It is sad that so often this has to be a substitute for human physical contact now so liable to be misunderstood in a perverse generation.

I had already completed this section on exercise, based mainly on case histories collected over the years, when there appeared in the *Daily Mail* advance excerpts from a then forthcoming book entitled *The Exercise Myth* under the heading 'the most controversial book on exercise for years'. This endorsed what I had long believed. For those who want to read more of the case against the self-inflicted consequences of unwisely strenuous exercise, and the advantages of truly regular and wisely adopted exercise, I commend this book, which some are already saying has 'the wisdom of Solomon'.

How marvellously is the mind improved by activity and motion of the body.

PLINY THE ELDER (A.D. 23-79).

REFERENCE

Dr Henry Solomon, *The Exercise Myth* (Angus & Robertson 1985).

Kenneth Vickery, 'Make Them Use Their Legs' *(Family Doctor* Sep 1962).

I I

Mind and Matter

The influence of the mind upon health, upon falling ill and upon recovery has been received knowledge since ancient times and the subject of profound pronouncement by the medical philosophers of old. It is perhaps as well that it has. Had it been a more recent observation we should probably be waiting for a randomized, controlled, double-blind trial before being able to make any use of this association, which derives much more from simple observation than scientific experiment.

A sound mind

There is a continuing 'chicken and egg' debate as to which is the dominant influence. Whichever, if either, comes first it is doubtful if there can be any such entity as a purely mental or purely physical disease. Certainly the association has been powerfully manipulated for evil, or for good, by witch-doctors and medicine-men and is never far from the practice of the wise physician.

Where manifestations of apparent mental ill-health predominate there can be no adequate assessment or treatment without full regard to the underlying physical state. And yes, predictably I say it again, close consideration of the food profile. Brain and nervous tissue is highly susceptible to deficiencies and contaminants in the fluids which bathe and nourish the delicate cells. Vital electrical responses can be impaired by mineral deficiency.

It is essential for every mother, every developing embryo, every baby, toddler and child, every mature adult, every elderly person to receive a flow of whole fresh nutrients sufficient in all requisite vital factors and trace elements, especially the B and E vitamins. Through this, mental deficiency and spina-bifida can be reduced; post-natal, pre-menstrual and endogenous depression abated; fractiousness and hyperactivity in children controlled; juvenile delinquency and criminal behaviour for kicks reduced. A host of conditions like schizophrenia and manic depressive psychosis can be abated, prevented and treated. The mental afflictions of old age may be diminished. The potential benefits of less stress and tension on accident rates, family violence and broken homes can be enjoyed.

All these desperately needed benefits have been observed repeatedly over the years, but because, on the whole, they have not lent themselves to controlled experiment, they are not respectably prescribable by the health professions. Yet anyone responsible for feeding a family, a communal residence, or a prison can put it to the test. Stated in reverse the most effective prescription for a maximum of delinquency, stroppiness and violence in an institution, is to give food consisting largely of refined white cereal in the form of bread, cakes, puddings, pastries loaded with sugar, hamburgers, sausages, vegetables overcooked in salt and bicarbonate, and a minimum of fresh element.

Not all in the mind

Closely linked with the deficiencies are the consequences of intolerance to individual foods, additives or contaminants in the environment. The generality of these intolerances has already been referred to but some of the worst of them surface as suspected mental illness. Hence the relevance of Dr Mackarness' *Not All in the Mind* and *Chemical Victims*. And if anyone should know, a psychiatrist should. But he also suffered from the 'not proven' verdict and left Britain for Australia where his efforts were to be better appreciated. I felt moved to say in a Foreword to the latter book that there are few more frustrating experiences in life than to feel persistently unwell, to be suffering from very real and even disabling symptoms, to be given a routine series of investigations by your GP and a specialist, only to be assured that nothing organically wrong has been found. You are expected to feel better and forget all about it, and if you don't, you're in real danger of being referred to a psychiatrist and becoming subject to his fearsome weapons.

There is a spate of illness, wrongly assumed to be psychiatric, which is in fact biochemical in origin, arising from nutritional deficiency, imbalance or sensitivity to food, combinations of food or chemicals, or medicinal drugs (prescribed or unprescribed). It has been very sad indeed to be aware of a number of these essentially preventable conditions treated by electro-convulsive therapy or powerful psychotropic drugs.

Freud, one of the founding fathers of modern psychiatry, was convinced that simple causes, related to bodily function, would one day be found for the greater part of all mental illness. It now surely makes sense, where vague, transient or inconsistent symptoms of mental illness are manifest to instruct the patient to persevere with a food reform diet and/or an elimination process to exclude food and chemical allergy.

Tension and stress

At the same time, physician and patient need to be aware of the possible cause, or influence, of undue stress and how we react to it on any illness. Unlike the insufficient understanding of the influence of food on health, the subject of stress, the emotional tensions engendered, and ways of coping with it, have been generally very well explained to the public. It has for years been an engaging subject for radio, TV and publications. Man now readily understands the results of his transposition from pastoral, rural, agrarian living (all in the space of a few recent years) to a noisy, polluted concrete jungle, surrounded and beset by teeming masses of people. He has taken the point that argument, anger and anxiety cause his muscles to tense and his glands to flood his bloodstream with the same hormones as his ancestors required to take flight, enter into physical combat or other strenuous physical activity. He is not surprised to be informed that there may be a price to be paid for frustrated hormonal response.

Nature's wonderful inbuilt powers of adaptation have been geared to a pace of change measured in terms of thousands of years and we are by no means yet adequately adapted to urban living. The big change which has occurred so rapidly and recently is in the kinds of stress now being encountered and in the increased frequency of our exposure. The stress of olden days tended to be severe and life threatening. It is evident for instance from a Victorian churchyard that at least half of the children born did not reach maturity. Countless mothers died in childbirth and it was quite usual for one or both parents to be dead by the age of forty-five. Premature death and illness caused tremendous hardship and real stress to the family.

By contrast, many of today's stresses, such as fighting the clock to keep appointments, finding a parking place and having noisy neighbours, must be regarded as trivial. But their continual impact, accelerated by relentless population expansion, causes a greater liability to symptoms of emotional tension than was manifest in our forefathers. Closely related is the markedly higher incidence of violence, crime, drug addiction and suicide in the cities.

Escapism

Man senses instinctively that the concrete jungle is not his natural habitat, and goes to considerable lengths to create little havens of wildlife and greenery under most unpromising conditions. He makes the most of his small backyard gardens, patios and window boxes. He has trailing plants and tropical fish in his home and office. At weekends and on holiday he will endure miles of surburban sprawl and slow-moving traffic for as little as a picnic in a green field or wood by the water. As he prospers in the city he will devote a significant proportion of his income to commuting daily from what is left of the country around his towns. The height of his ambition may be a weekend country cottage further out.

Mercifully this urge to get away from it all, and be apart from time to time, is therapeutic—as our Lord well knew. So too is the desire to grow and eat home produce, to keep goats, poultry and bees and to make bread with motivation often way ahead of economic necessity. Man yearns for the 'good life' and his TV programme makers and advertisers are well aware of it.

Emotions which boomerang

Emotions which can be a great source of distress, sorrow, despair and danger to those about us include anger, rage, temper, hatred, jealousy, resentment, unforgiveness, selfish ambition and a revengeful spirit. Whatever the effect on others, and it may be little or great, the most certain and unrelenting consequences are upon ourselves. In the short term or long term these emotions, sustained or repeated, turn back on us and become a most powerful precipitating factor in physical and mental illness. Likewise anxiety, fear and guilt exact a similar heavy toll. A law-abiding householder for instance may be convinced, with every justification and evidence, that a neighbour has repositioned the boundary posts and unjustly acquired a small slice of his land. If the injured party responds to this situation with constant heated argument, resentment, prolonged lawsuit or retaliation he can make himself ill and shorten his life considerably. A vastly greater cost than the value of the land. The possible cost to health has to be weighed even where the injury is far greater.

Early symptoms of excessive emotion include nausea, vomiting, loss of appetite, headache, irregular heart-beat, skin rash, wheezing and over-breathing. Fully blown illnesses so precipitated can include high blood pressure, coronary thrombosis, stroke, rheumatism, asthma, alcoholism, arthritis and peptic ulcer. To be aware of these risks of self-inflicted backlash is important; many remain ignorant that their emotions and behavioural responses could possibly have any effect upon health. Yet the fact is that chemical changes take place in the body whether the emotions be harmful or beneficial.

For true effective mastery of the illness-causing consequences of unbridled emotions there is only one course: a transformation by the renewing of the mind.

Many people today, when seen by the doctor, feel that they have been cheated if he omits to write them out a prescription for medicine. Whereas so often (though it may cost him much more effort) the prescription really needed is considered advice, directed to substantial changes in the way of life. The necessary alterations in lifestyle, which must be ongoing, demand efforts of will which unaided are so often beyond the resolve of the patient to sustain. Consciously or subconsciously he knows this, which is why he continues to hope that there may be an alternative such as the latest wonder drug to calm his emotions, his mood swings, his unbridled appetites and his recurrent depression.

Divine prescriptions

It is right here at the heart of mental health that the unfailing answer is to be found. The words of the Master and his servants presented in Scripture are not only the prescription but carry the promise of power to enable the prescription to be effective. The invitation is to 'be transformed by the renewing of your mind' (Romans 12:2, NIV). The key to this prescription, which is the antidote to the disease-producing emotions, is to be found in our Lord's New Testament confirmation of the greatest commandment in the law given by God through Moses. This is to 'love the Lord your God with all your heart, and with all your soul and with all your mind'. The closely related second is to 'love your neighbour as yourself' (Matthew 22:37-39, NIV).

The seemingly difficult injunction to love and pray for those who abuse us, has proven in practice to be a protective healing balm to the abused and epitomizes a most significant difference between the Christian faith and any other religion. Noting also that we are required to love our neighbour *as* ourself. Not more than, not less than, and not instead of. Self-deprecation, feelings of excessive unworthiness, self-despising, self-hatred and self-pity—especially self-pity—are hindrances to sound mental health. It is not a required Christian virtue to refrain from a healthy sufficiency of self-esteem.

The Scriptures are rich in supplementary prescriptions for sound mental health. The following are particularly worthy of heed: 'Now you must rid yourselves of all such things as these: anger, rage, malice, slander and filthy language' (Colossians 3:8, NIV); and 'Fret not thyself' (Psalm 37:7).

Selwyn Hughes (acknowledged in chapter 14), expressing views endorsed by many doctors, maintains that our attitudes have a tremendous and powerful influence on every part of our being. He concludes that the eight principles which comprise the beatitudes are the best prescription for mental and spiritual health that it is possible to find (Matthew 5:1-11).

Also on the positive side we have that tremendous prescription of St Paul regarding the right feeding of the mind as essential to mental health:

> Whatsoever things are true, whatsoever things are honest, whatsoever things are just, whatsoever things are pure, whatsoever things are lovely, whatsoever things are of good report; if there be any virtue, and if there be any praise, think on these things (Philippians 4:8).

The message of divine wisdom cries out from the Scriptures that there is bad food and good food for the mind and that a man *is* how he thinks.

And we arrive at another remarkable analogy between food for the body and food for the mind. We have seen how, in the case of food in its related illness, the unthinking, the unheeding, the unobservant and those of vested interest fall back on the cliches of 'insufficient scientific evidence' or 'not proven'. We have the same negative lobby in the case of food for the mind.

A minority of the observant, concerned and responsible can see with frightening clarity the consequences of a daily and nightly diet of violence, murder, rape, terrorism, sexual depravity, mugging, blackmail, strife, envy, greed, exploitation, abuse and lawlessness vividly displayed on the screen. They see only too clearly the connection between the rising tide of crime and its explicit example on TV and video—added to by pornography in literature and on stage. Yet what is the loud rejoinder whenever a warning cry is uttered? 'There is no convincing evidence of any association between fiction and crime.' And neither were the prophets heard, even during the last days of the decline and fall of Rome and other great empires.

Fear not

Fear of what might befall us is an emotion which can take a heavy toll upon health—especially in these perilous times. Indeed we are warned in the Bible of times when men's hearts are failing them for fear of what is coming on the world. Yet beautifully and paradoxically the antidote to worldly fear is fear of the Lord stemming from appreciation of his power and love towards man and fostering in us the will towards obedience. So we read and appreciate that 'Perfect love casteth out fear' (1 John 4:18), and that the Lord will bless them that fear him and be their help and shield (Psalm 115).

'Be still and know' (Psalm 46:10)

This divine prescription is reiterated throughout Scripture. Expressed in Psalm 37:7 it is, 'Rest in the Lord and wait patiently for him.' We are left in no doubt that periods of rest are necessary for man's mind and body. Our Lord found it essential to be by himself from time to time and commended his disciples to do likewise. The principle of the Sabbath as a day of rest for spiritual refreshment is enshrined in the Ten

Commandments.

The wisdom of relaxation and meditation is not exclusively biblical. Its importance has been recognized and practised in the orient for millennia. The essential ingredients of posture, movement, mental control and breathing control are all vital. Christians can derive the physical and mental benefits with the added bonus of the meditation being biblical, prayerful and positive. Secular and oriental chants and incantations must be rejected. Reams and volumes have been written on the essentials of the techniques, but suffice it here just to say that conscious relaxation is an essential adjuvant to health.

Biofeedback

It is of interest to add that out of this appreciation of the importance of learning how to relax, man has been able to harness electro-instrumental means to monitor degrees of relaxation and to assist in furthering it. I refer to the biofeedback devices, some now freely available and relatively inexpensive, which can enable the subject to monitor his degree of relaxation and to help him to improve it. In reality such machines prove what has long been suspected by a minority: that man, by effort of will, can gain a measure of control over such an essentially involuntary function as the level of his blood pressure. Some might call it 'mind over matter'.

I am not suggesting that access to a biofeedback instrument is necessary or desirable. It is the case, however, that a part of the same technology which spawns high-speed living can be applied to defuse some of the stress consequences of its jet lag.

Sleep—nature's restorative balm

I find it very difficult to accept any explanation of the phenomenon of sleep other than that of a divine restorative provision for man and wildlife. Those who are deprived of sleep through illness or circumstances add to the testimony of how dearly this gift should be prized. The facility to sleep in peace and dwell in safety is gratefully acknowledged by man in Psalm 4:8 and 127:2.

To assist in claiming the benefits of sleep we are urged not to worry about tomorrow (Matthew 6:34) and commanded not to let the sun go down on our wrath (Ephesians 4:26). We are reminded over and over again of the restorative power of prayer, particularly prayer in the evening when the unresolved concerns of the day are laid before the Lord. At a more secular level it is common experience for the unconscious mind to solve problems by the morning. For the Christian there is a deeper and more profound ministry in sleep. When we pray for wisdom and discernment it is very often in sleep that the Holy Spirit prepares us for wise counsel in the day ahead.

Cancer, the precipitating and the healing factors

I have already referred (in chapter 2) to the importance of nutritional wholeness as the best possible means of enabling the body to resist disease of all kinds, with particular reference to cancer. Observational evidence continues to convince me that the underlying cause of most cancer is nutritional deficiency.

The riddle of what loads the dice has been pertinently expressed in *World Medicine* of London:

> One of the great injustices of life on earth—or anyway in the West—is the way some people can stuff their lungs and guts with carcinogens from the age of 12 and still live to 90 whereas others pay the penalty in late middle age.

The body is dependent upon its nutritional state to resist the many and repeated environmental assaults upon it. When all is well, damaged tissues are continually repaired which, as has been said, is the essence of God's provision of healing. When the body's nutritional state is impoverished, the cells are increasingly liable to become disorderly in the face of such inflictions as natural or man-made radiation, smoking, atmospheric pollution, food contaminants and additives, excess alcohol or that small number of cancer types induced by viruses. All these and more are precipitating factors but their part in no way justifies calling cancer a disease of multiple causes. One of the most powerful precipitating factors is regarded by many to be the psychological. This factor is so real that valid 'photofits' have been constructed of cancer personalities—people with a higher than average chance of getting cancer.

Features of the cancer personality-type include persistent feelings of inadequacy, deferred hopes, unworthiness and dislike of self—particularly if these things stem from the lack of satisfactory parental relationships. Included in these features is an inability to express justifiable emotions while maintaining an appearance of long suffering, goodness and kindness, and frustrated outlet for talents and abilities.

Given such a personality and state, the last straw unleashing cancer, which may have been incubating for many years, can so often be an event of bereavement such as loss of a life partner, broken marriage, divorce or family tragedy, with guilt and depression in attendance.

Whole person medicine

The recognition of the reality of these cancer-provoking factors has paved the way for long-overdue perception of cancer in relation to the whole person. Some now give attention to the physical, emotional and spiritual implications which contributed to its onset with a view to harnessing their positive potential to combat the disease. Relaxation and mental imagery have proved to be powerful positive forces—for instance, visualizing the body's natural healing systems mopping up rogue cancer cells—as indeed occurs throughout life. This approach has found pioneer and promising expression in the UK at the Bristol Cancer Help Centre—the subject of a TV documentary which aroused considerable interest. Nevertheless America was at least ten years ahead of us in appreciation of some aspects of the approach.

The philosophy of the Bristol work has been perceptively written up in *A Gentle Way with Cancer*. When in the early eighties a centre was established with the backing and participation of qualified doctors and other members of the health professions I was extremely heartened. Predictably I would rejoice that fundamental to the entire approach was restoration by means of whole fresh food. This is based partly on attention to the kinds of foods eaten by races found to be remarkably free from cancer and the preventive and healing properties of the kernels of the fruits. Apricot kernels in particular direct attention to the special vitamins found at the heart of the concentrated wonders of nature's new growth. Here at last in Britain the essence of Bircher-Benner's raw food therapies, whose continuing benefits had been demonstrated for at least half a century, were being combined in a holistic approach enlisting the active participation of the patient to contribute to the process of healing. Amen to that!

The beauty of the 'gentle way' is that it is not only Alternative Medicine. It can be very helpful Supplementary Medicine (taken with the knowledge and co-operation of the patient's doctor) where surgery and/or chemotherapy and radiotherapy have been undertaken. Even in the absence of an understanding doctor it is the entitlement of every individual to choose his food wisely along the lines of the Bristol diet, and cultivate positive mental attitudes to health and healing. No possible harm can result and thousands can testify to much benefit.

The heartrending decision as to whether early or advanced cancer patients should place entire reliance on the 'gentle way', or have the dedication to persevere, are dealt with in the book. Nothing I say here, or elsewhere, must be construed as incitement to go against the advice of the family physician. I would say, however, that for anyone who harbours morbid fear of cancer, is visiting or nursing a relative or friend with cancer, or who is suffering from cancer and has sought medical advice, the book can be nothing but helpful. Not least for those who do not have cancer and wish to follow an unworried way of life, reducing the possibilities of contracting it.

Meanwhile, more orthodox research continues apace. There is now a tremendous fund of knowledge on cell biology, genetic abnormalities, vulnerable genes, mutations, the mechanisms of immunity and the beneficial antibodies. Man will continue his search for the treatment of cancer, the elixir whereby he need not submit to the discipline of healthy ways of living. But that time is not yet. Meanwhile, nature continues with her consequences.

Alternative Medicine

This may be an appropriate point to say a little more about this subject even though the systems, cults and therapies now collectively embraced in the term are by no means exclusively of the mind. They include homeopathy, acupuncture, reflexology, herbalism, osteopathy, chiropraxis and naturopathy.

The temptation for the patient to depart from the orthodox is at its greatest whenever a verdict is given of 'nothing further can be done'. Many claims to success have been made over the years by practitioners and patients. Certain established factors can account for at least some of them. The first is enthusiasm and a new approach. Many unorthodox therapies pursued with confidence by healer and patient will have a success rate. Some successes will be related to the 'placebo effect', that is, a proportion of patients in trials with new drugs will improve when given an inert substance of the same appearance as the medicine to be tested.

It is quite usual for practitioners of Alternative Medicine to spend more time in personal discussion with the patient than doctors usually find possible. It is also more common for the patient to be made to be personally involved in the treatment: self-health.

One way to become acquainted with the range and scope of Alternative Medicine is to visit one of the annual conventions. There can be found under one roof stands and exhibitions featuring most of the many movements. Keeping eyes and ears open as one walks around, it is evident that many people who attend are seeking a solution to their problems. Accordingly, to meet this demand Alternative Medicine, as its very name suggests, is scarcely less preoccupied with treatment and cure than is the orthodox. It must be admitted, however, that more encouragement is given towards healthy habits of living, particularly in the matter of food. Much of the thinking in Alternative Medicine sees the wisdom of attention to the whole person. This includes recognition of the spiritual dimension in health and life. No small part of this is, unfortunately, appropriated by the non-Christian cults, gurus, pundits, mystics, oriental meditators and astrologers. The Christian commitment to sound spiritual and mental health is much less well manifested. We do well to remember the void within each one of us which longs to be filled by the Holy Spirit.

There are some components of Alternative Medicine, such as naturopathy and osteopathy, that I would like to see represented in our health centres and group medical practices. This would involve an enlargement of the health team, and a working together of the practitioners within agreed guidelines, thus enabling the busy doctor, after counselling the patient, to delegate the health education, alternative remedial/ medical treatment to the other members of the team. In this way the 'whole' patient may be understood and catered for. In such a setting the term Complementary Medicine is much to be preferred. All of this will need to be preceded by the adoption of recognized standards of training and competence of the complementary practitioners.

There is a wide, almost bewildering, brash of health magazines extolling the alternatives. The better end of these can be soundly helpful on whole, fresh and live food, weight control, relaxation, breathing and tempered exercise. The down-market end of the magazines can be unjustifiably scathing of orthodox medicine. They may also be unwisely overdedicated to fitness through excessive exercise, and may carry advertisements making specious claims in the matter of food supplements and suggestions of dubious propriety in such matters as rejuvenation and the improvement of flagging sexual vigour.

What cannot be ignored is the very considerable public interest in Alternative Medicine, particularly among this generation. It is evident from the media and personal contact that there are many people prepared to testify glowingly to having received profound help who had no relief from orthodox medicine.

The British Medical Association aware of this public interest has recently, following deliberation, issued a report which received a very bad press. Much of the press comment, rather unfairly, centred around what the report had to say about homeopathy. Nevertheless I have the feeling that doctors of this generation will be much less inhibited in referring their patients to such as non-medically qualified osteopaths and naturopaths than were their predecessors.

Beware the unholy spirits

I conclude this chapter on a cautionary note, referring again to that void within all of us which God longs to fill. It is essential to ensure that when the mind is relaxed and emptied by any of the means mentioned, it is filled only with prayerful, uplifting thoughts. If this is not positively encouraged there is risk of the void being filled with the spirits of evil. The Bible leaves us in no doubt of their existence. Such is the spiritual hunger of man, it is tragically easy to be seduced into spiritism, witchcraft and other devices of satanism. Counterfeit miracles can reach into the realms of healing and deceive even the elect. Man is expressly warned in Scripture against dabbling in the occult—specifically in Leviticus 20:6, Deuteronomy 18:9-14 and Acts 8:9-24; 13:6-12. The penalty was, and is, a considerable risk of mental illness through demonization. The promise of safety in the face of all these and other assaults is typified in Psalm 91: 'There shall no evil befall thee.'

Discernment in health and healing comes through opening the door to the Holy Spirit.

For God hath not given us the spirit of fear; but of power, and of love, and of a sound mind.

2 Timothy 1:7.

REFERENCE

Brenda Kidman, *A Gentle Way With Cancer* (Century 1985).
Richard Mackarness, *Not All in the Mind* (Pan Books 1976).
Richard Mackarness, *Chemical Victims* (Pan Books 1980).
Miranda Robertson, 'Cancer: What loads the dice?' *(World Medicine* Vol.18 no.20 1983).

12

Apostles of Health

. . . in science the credit goes to the man who convinces the world, not to the man to whom the idea first occurs.
Sir Francis Darwin (1914).

Society owes a very considerable debt to a small number of enlightened people who, over the past 100 years or so, have been pioneers in challenging public and professional opinion to appreciate that unhealthy habits of food production and consumption are the biggest single cause of mankind's enormous burden of degenerative disease. I've called them 'apostles of health' which is no disrespect to the biblical use of the term 'holy apostles' and those who qualify for this description.

I find that little previous attempt has been made to honour or link these names together. I feel this should be attempted in order to teach us something of the ecological and multi-disciplinary approach necessary for the understanding of health. Inevitably any such citation will be imperfect and somewhat dependent upon a compiler's nationality, profession and prejudices. It is remarkable though that even give or take a few, the number of true pioneers of health only amounts to the tiniest fraction of the thousands of those who would be listed as having made signal contributions to the study of disease and its treatment.

Some parts of my reference to these pioneers is intended to illustrate the way ahead. It is interesting to note that among these people is the common denominator of arriving at a minority view and standing fast in the face of apathy, ridicule, vested interest and deferred career prospect. There is consistent humility in their approach and a sense of awe at the wonders of nature. Most significant of all, as evident from their utterances and writings, is that a high proportion are on record as practising Christians who acknowledge their God as the great Creator and Architect of the universe, and the inspiration of their work. I have been most impressed while mulling through the writings of the apostles of health to find how timeless and up-to-date their message remains. By contrast the textbooks on disease and treatment seem out-of-date almost before they leave the press. The manifestations of disease are changing, restless and so often at least one jump ahead of the efforts to cure, but the principles of health are unchanging.

Claims that one or other of the pioneers of health was the first to use or draw attention to some such measures as a dietary reform should be assessed with great caution. Twentieth-century pioneers may be credited for persisting with the case for wholefood and raw food and against excess refined carbohydrate, but they were preceded by earlier advocates. For some years I was conscious that the Seventh Day Adventists had been decades ahead of their time in their health education activity to these ends. I later became aware that an American adventist sect known as 'The Shakers' practised a wholefood way of life in their closed communities some 200 years ago.

The length of the following citations and their order of mention is in no way intended to denote any assessment of relative merit.

Dr Thomas Richard Allinson

We begin with this worthy name, well known in the cause of food reform. Allinson qualified with honours in medicine in 1879 but eschewed fashionable practice for work as a parish doctor in London's east end. Ill-health abounded. He quickly perceived that, along with poverty, the biggest cause was poor food. He encouraged his patients and their families towards simple, inexpensive, wholegrain foods. He singled out bread for particular attention. He persuaded some hundreds of bakers to produce wholewheat loaves according to his recipe, and awarded them certificates for display. In spite of his self-less life his jealous enemies dubbed him a crank and a char-latan. They succeeded in getting him struck off the medical register on the pretext of self-advertisement. Judging from the cartoons of the time his detractors, who were ridiculed as bigots, came off worst. He truly deserves to be remembered as the patron saint of 'wholemeal'.

Taunted by the 'scientific proof' brigade Allinson devised a biological experiment. He arranged to subsist for a month on water and simple unleavened wholemeal loaves, resembling the oriental chapatti. He completed the course in full vigour carrying on his busy active work. By way of controls a well-known dietitian and an assistant began under the same con-ditions with white bread. They had to give up within three weeks having been overcome by malaise and weakness. His critics did not admit to being impressed.

One who *was* impressed with Allinson's work was Mahatma Gandhi, then a law student in London. On return to India he was much preoccupied with food, poverty and health, and he wrote a book called *Food Reform*.

Allinson's work of education and food reform went from strength to strength. He took over a stone-mill in 1892 to safeguard his bakers against the adulterated coloured white flour then prevalent. The business prospered as the Natural Food Company, then later as Allinson Ltd—of which one of his sons became director. Happily and deservedly the name of Allinson has lived to see wholemeal bread, at long last, the preferred bread of the discerning public and endorsed by a consensus of the health professions.

Sir Albert Howard

Albert Howard's work was mostly in India from the early part of this century. His significant contribution was to understanding soil—the foundation of physical life. He saw the soil as a living organism and sought to ensure that all the available organic waste of civilized life was returned to it. He recognized the ancient wisdom of the Chinese in hastening the breakdown process and preparing the resultant humus away from the field. He was the founding father of applied composting. He also had to kick against the pricks of officialdom.

Most valuable of all his works were the carefully controlled experiments revealing the relationship between healthy soil and healthy crops with resistance to disease, and between healthy animals and healthy crops. He had the vision to see the wholeness of this cycle and relate to it the health of man. Truly he also was a master of ecology. But many wasted years were to elapse before even half-hearted acceptance of his principles was made.

Sir Robert McCarrison

Working at much the same time (1902-35) and also in India was Robert McCarrison. To him goes the credit of recording the state of health and disease of respective races on the Indian continent as being directly related to the quality of the food. It was he who told the world of the exceptionally fine health of the Hunza related to their basic diet of freshly ground wholewheat flour made into loaves of unleavened bread, along with milk, butter, curds, fresh vegetables, fruit and occasional meat. This contrasted starkly with the poor health and poor diet of the Madrassis and their like. He also carried out a quite unique form of animal feeding experiment. Having observed the state of health of the races in relation to their food, he reproduced the same health patterns in colonies of rats by feeding them the racial diets. He thus turned white-mouse medicine on its head most laudably. To him we owe the dictum: 'The greatest single factor in the acquisition and maintenance of good health is perfectly constituted food.'

Deservedly his name is perpetuated by the McCarrison Society founded as a forum for doctors, dentists and veterinary scientists to pursue their common and interdisciplinary interests in the influence of nutrition in health and disease. It is also right to couple with his name that of Dr Hugh M. Sinclair, Fellow of Magdalen College, Oxford, who has devoted his professional life to the integrity of nutrition and carried the torch of McCarrison's work into the latter half of the twentieth century.

Weston A. Price MS DDS

If one exploration of health more than another could be described as the most blindly neglected piece of vital research of all time, it is the research undertaken by American dental surgeon Weston Price. Commencing in the early thirties he found some fifty isolated communities worldwide and contrasted their dental condition and general health with similar races having access to sophisticated modern food. As he travelled along trade routes he found dental disease decreasing and eventually when he passed the last trading post he found people who were dependent on their own economy and remarkably free from disease. He was able to contrast them with peoples from the same communities who had left the tribe to subsist where commercial sophisticated food was available.

These pre-Second World War journeys were made in the nick of time. There are few of these primitive races left today. He found that primitive peoples subsisted on unrefined, whole, unprocessed and fresh foods. He brought back photographic evidence of their fine teeth, healthy gums, perfect dental arches and handsome facial form. They also manifested marked freedom from degenerative disease generally and were by and large happy and contented people.

In sharp contrast, one generation of sugary, refined commercial food sufficed to cause them to lose their fine teeth, physique, stamina and morale. They became morose, discontented and quarrelsome—a finding which has also been mirrored in colonies of rats.

The statement of Price most deserving of immortality is: 'Food is fabricated soil fertility.' I can think of no one in his time more deserving of a posthumous Nobel Prize. I would like to feel that had the 1966 scientific reappraisals of the Foundation taken place twenty years earlier he might have been so honoured.

Max O. Bircher-Benner

If the observations and teachings of this Swiss doctor, which were fully available more than half a century ago, had been acknowledged millions of lives could have been physically and mentally transformed. It was he, along with his medically qualified family, who established the essentials of a whole, fresh, substantially uncooked diet—the self same diet which the so-called 'supernutritionists' are pleading for today. The same diet which is implicit in today's 'gentle ways' with cancer. The principles of healthy eating which he worked out in the early days of this century require no alteration to this day. He is best remembered for his Swiss Bircher muesli or raw fruit porridge.

Thomas Latimer Cleave FRCP Surg. Capt. RN

Outstanding as an observer and thinker, Cleave was among the few who got to the heart of the matter of promoting health and preventing disease in the mid-twentieth century. It has been suggested that the essence of his contribution, without which this book could not be complete, is encompassed at both secular and spiritual levels by the words of thanksgiving I was privileged to give in his honour (some of which are reproduced opposite). I had simultaneously been given the opportunity in writing *The Times* obituary to refer to some of the conditions embraced in his concept of the Saccharine Disease.

Cleave's work is central to my wider concept of Deplete Food Disease. I am deeply grateful for his original thinking.

Extracts from the
Thanksgiving for the life work of
SURGEON CAPTAIN THOMAS LATIMER CLEAVE
23rd Sept. 1983

The praise of man in the House of God is not to be undertaken lightly. However, some of us who knew Peter Cleave over the years saw so many things working together for good, to have no doubt, that his life's work should be interpreted as contributing to the will and glory of God. . . .

Peter was profoundly moved by the premature death of a young sister . . . from acute appendicitis and later of his mother, following much suffering. A medical commission in the Royal Navy, during which he prepared himself for higher qualifications, provided him with a unique opportunity to contrast disease findings of Western culture, with those of more primitive societies, wherever his ship took him—worldwide, in the laboratory of nature.

He discerned that the key to the patterns of health and disease observed was the nature of the food taken, and the biggest single factor in the food was the degree of refinement of cereal, rice and sugar plants.

Naval life, particularly during World War II also provided opportunities for observing ships' companies captive to available diet, which was the same opportunity which led to James Lind's memorable work on scurvy. But it was yet to be many long years before consensus medical opinion would be prepared to accept these kinds of epidemological evidence as a basis for health education towards change. However, his abilities were not unappreciated by the Senior Service, who appointed him Director of Medical Research.

Way back in the post-war fifties Peter and I, who had no previous acquaintance, experienced one of those remarkable simultaneous events which the world calls 'coincidence'. Out of the blue we posted letters of encouragement to one another on the very same day. From that time forward, and for some thirty years, I was privileged to sharpen my wits upon his superb intellect. He had little time for small talk and social gatherings, but he could be charming, with a fine sense of humour, and his company always stimulating, especially in his observation of the world of nature.

His period in the professional wilderness was all of 40 years, during which he suffered ridicule, incredulity and open hostility, but Peter was successively brought into contact with other enquiring minds, some also kicking against the pricks, who were a considerable professional encouragement to him—and whose findings contrived to forging further links in his wide hypothesis. At the end of the road, it was a Christian doctor, already distinguished in another field, whose support in the later seventies was more than anything responsible for the consensus medical acceptance of substantial parts of Peter's work.

His Royal Highness Prince Charles, in his recent Presidential Address to the British Medical Association referred to the deeply ingrained suspicion and outright hostility which can exist towards the unorthodox and unconventional. He went on to say—and I quote—'Perhaps we have to accept it is God's will that the unorthodox individual is doomed to years of frustration, ridicule and failure, in order to act out his role in the scheme of things, until his day arrives, and mankind is ready to receive his message—a message which he probably finds hard to explain, but which he knows comes from a far deeper source than conscious thought.'

These inspired words could have been tailor-made for Peter Cleave, whose ancestor, Bishop Hugh Latimer, died in the flames for propagating obstinate ideas which were inconvenient to the establishment.

As Peter was only too well aware, the composition of the wheat berry, in its wholeness of vital nutrients, vitamins, minerals and trace elements is a sermon in itself. It is ironic that the breakthrough of the acceptance of Peter's work eventually came from the hitherto least valued and most discarded fraction of the wheat, the bran—never, until lately, restored when they tried to rebuild white flour so grievously impoverished by the mills. Bran of the husks that the swine did eat. The stone that the builders' rejected. Hopefully, history will yet accept Peter's own priority that even the bran is not the most significant part of his work, which is in fact sugar and over-consumption facilitated by refinement.

The obituaries have dealt with his many gifts and talents; ornithology, linguistics, fly fishing, and with his most readable and best-selling books, culminating with the Saccharine Disease, and with his summons, years before recognition in his own country to give evidence before the U.S. Senate Select Committee. His subsequent election to the Fellowship of the Royal College of Physicians and, happiest day of all, in his beloved Haslar Hospital in 1979, the simultaneous presentation of two gold medals by the Royal Colleges and the Royal Institute of Public Health in the presence of his Naval medical colleagues and others eminent in the field of nutrition.

Denis Burkitt MD FRCS FRS

It has been said that the most powerful obstacle to progress is a new idea. It is certainly true in medical and scientific circles that reception of a new idea is closely related to the academic status of the proponent. However brilliant a concept, if the advocate is relatively unknown its progress will have a hard time. Allinson and Cleave knew what it was to experience this.

In marked contrast, when Denis Burkitt began in the seventies to draw attention to the public health implications of the refining of food and dietary fibre he received a much more immediate hearing. He was at pains to give due acknowledgement to the earlier work and writings of Cleave, but had previously made his name in discovering a cancer tumour among the Africans. This was just the kind of disease discovery beloved of the scientific establishment. They gave his name to it: Burkitt's lymphoma. And a more than well-deserved honour that it should be so, for this Christian doctor spent years of painstaking observation under primitive conditions across wide tracts of Africa. His eventual findings were a blessing to the child sufferers of this malignant disease. But his greatest benefit to mankind was to arise from endorsing this same kind of observational research in the field of Western diet deficiencies, and being listened to. It would be difficult not to see the hand of God in this. His fascinating life story has been written up by Brian Kellock.

Burkitt's crucial part is a further illustration of sociologist Robert Merton's phenomenon 'the Matthew effect' ('unto everyone that hath shall be given . . .' [Matthew 25:29]).

And all praise to Burkitt. Even he had had to put up with ridicule for sharing common ground with cranks while he persuaded a sceptical profession to appreciate the importance of the consistency, size and floatability of the human stool, and something as despised and unspectacular as bran.

Sir William Arbuthnot Lane Bart.

I promised in chapter 1 a further mention of Sir William. He certainly deserves it, and to be regarded as the patron saint of health education. His entitlement to that honour stems first from a brilliant clinical career. Lane goes down in history as one of the most versatile and distinguished surgeons of all time.

His surgical skill was attracted to the major contemporary problems of his times. Prominent among these, and at its height during the first decade of the twentieth century, was intractable chronic constipation. Constipation which was so severe that it seemed necessary to resort to the surgeon's knife to relieve it, as we have seen with the bishop's wife.

He performed many of these colectomy operations, but we note that he became increasingly aware that constipation was mostly preventable. He was clearly saddened at having to perform the operation, and notwithstanding his personal high success rate, the inevitable failures grieved him.

Constipation under the description of intestinal stasis, provoked endless debate in the medical societies. Lane encountered great opposition to his predictions of its baleful consequences, including cancer. His thinking was years ahead of his time!

Constipation and his perceptive observation of its causes was undoubtedly the stimulus for the last chapter of his life. He reasoned that unless the public could be made aware of the faulty habits of living, which predisposed to many of the conditions of civilized life, there was no prospect of effective prevention.

With great courage in 1926 he laid down his scalpel and founded the New Health Society with the object of teaching people the simple laws of health; of promoting the consumption of whole cereals, fresh fruit and vegetables and encouraging people to go back to the land to relieve the overcrowding of towns and provide healthy gainful occupation and fresh food.

Lane, assisted by his wife, energetically threw himself into the educational activities of the New Health Society and journal. He found the public to be hungry for advice on healthy living. He steeled himself to undertake public lectures. Vast halls were filled to overflowing to hear him. The *Daily Mail* quickly saw the significance of a new public desire for health information, and articles by Lane were published. Remarkably, I recently found one which had been lining the bottom of an old family suitcase for sixty years.

He entered into public health education in the full knowledge that, although there was no possible personal gain (indeed the Society was a charge on his own resources), he would incur the displeasure of the medical profession and its so-called ethical committees. And so he did. There was much bitterness, with threats that he would be struck off the Medical Register. His attitude to this opposition was characterized by his stated opinion that if a man, having considered what is a right course of action, hesitates and wonders what people will say—that man will not attain anything worth while.

His response to his detractors was conditioned, as he put it, from his early biblical studies: 'Love your enemies and do good to them that despitefully use you'!

The notable honour in Lane's life, his baronetcy, derived from his surgical skills and shortly followed his successful operation on a Princess of the Royal House in 1913. But in order to fulfil what we can now see as his greatest work—preventive medicine—he felt it necessary to humble himself and hand back the most prized possession of a doctor, his place on the Medical Register of the General Medical Council.

It is sad indeed that as recently as 1933, when Lane requested the erasure of his name, our medical profession remained so hidebound and obtuse as to be unwilling to countenance a retired doctor, the essential meaning of whose title is 'teacher', performing his most valuable and selfless role so far as the suffering public was concerned. It is to the credit of some who recognized Lane's true worth that immediately prior to his voluntary erasure he was made a life-Fellow of the prestigious London Medical Society.

One is not aware of whether the British Medical Association ever relented. However, Lane's biographer notes with satisfaction that some ten years later the BMA's own Secretary, Dr Charles Hill, was conducting mass health education as the Radio doctor. Subsequently the BMA launched its own health education journal *Family Doctor* with signed articles written by doctors. Lane, however, would not have rejoiced at much of its content (mostly indifferent to food reform). The worst example, and a blatant and ignorant distortion of true health education, was the cover and supplement of the December 1959 edition. This flagrantly advocated lashings of sugar as a commended food for healthy living.

Doris Grant

Important as the discovery of the components of health is, it avails little unless the message is put over to the public.

Doris Grant is a worthy representative of the British teachers of living health. No one has written more consistently and persuasively for so long as Doris. She is quoted at length in Dr Lionel Picton's perceptive book *Thoughts on Feeding* written some forty years ago. This reveals that she was already active during the war years providing 'Victory Recipes' for wholemeal bread, wholewheat scones and fruit loaf. In the meantime she has written and sold many thousands of a wide range of purposeful and health-seeking books. Her early classic was *Your Daily Bread* in which she immortalized the labour-saving Grant loaf (see chapter 6). And her pen continues to be active as we move towards the nineties.

Everard Turner BDS

This most observant dental surgeon, and founder member of the Soil Association, appreciated that the tooth and state of the mouth was a window to the condition of all the tissues of the body. He pioneered the concept that poor teeth reflected much more than the sugar-laden food which daily afflicted their surfaces. The heart of the matter was somatic—the impoverished, lifeless food which failed to build up and maintain the tooth and jaw structure.

W.E. Shewell-Cooper MBE NDH FLS D.Litt

The late Dr Shewell-Cooper's contribution to the health of soil, plant, animal and man has been outstanding. All this he explored and taught in a Christian missionary context at his Thaxted Horticultural College and Arkley Manor gardens.

Neil S. Painter MS FRCS

Great credit is due to this surgeon of brilliant mind and Hunterian Professor of the Royal College of Surgeons who knowingly suffered hindrance to his surgical career in order to pursue research into bowel disease. His clinical trials in the early sixties have been of inestimable value to mankind in turning on its head the established treatment of diverticular disease and pointing the way to its prevention by the restoration of dietary fibre in Western food (see chapter 1).

Dr Lionel James Picton OBE

One of the most perceptive of British General Practitioners of all time. In 1939 he was able to encourage all thirty-two doctor members of the Cheshire Local Medical and Panel Committees, representing some 600 General Practitioners, to sign a most damning Medical Testament, deploring the state of the nation's health and indicting wrong nutrition as the major cause. Sadly the intervention of World War Two interrupted the momentum which this exposure might otherwise have gathered.

Lady Eve Balfour

She had the vision to collate together the relevance of the work of McCarrison, Howard, Picton and others. She was also the founding inspiration of the Soil Association in 1946, bringing together a wide variety of disciplines with regard to the health of plant, animal and man and their interdependence.

Dr Innes H. Pearse

We are indebted to her, along with her husband Dr G. Scott Williamson, for the founding of the Peckham Pioneer Health Centre for the studying of health and function in family context. This was an experiment sadly interrupted and curtailed by the consequences of World War Two, but one which pushed forward the frontiers of our knowledge of health.

Sir Francis Avery Jones CBE, MD, FRCP

A distinguished gastro-enterologist, always ahead of his time in his perception of the influence of personal habits of living and of commercial practices upon health and disease. His respect for natural principles was already manifest in the thirties and led him progressively to appreciate the preventive and healing potential of whole and fresh foods.

Maurice Frohn FRCS

He has contributed much to prevention, by dietary means, of

the dreaded post-operative deep-vein thrombosis and pulmonary thrombosis, and we are indebted to him for his splendid colour photography revealing at operation the mechanisms involved.

Conrad Latto FRCS

He continues with parallel research in his surgical wards on the prevention of disease and is a worthy representative of a medical family name to whom much is owed in the promotion of health.

Kenneth Heaton MD MRCP

A latter day pioneer pursuing necessary and painstaking research into the nature of foodstuff and their utilization by the body. He has added considerably to the knowledge of the nature of fibre and its function on ingestion, including the important role of satiety when meals are taken. He was mainly responsible, as honorary secretary, in recording and expressing the medical consensus which led to the Royal College of Physicians 1980 Report on Dietary Fibre.

Walter Yellowlees MC FRCGP

Much is owed to this observant Scottish General Practitioner for perceiving the true cause of the exceptionally high rate of disease and mortality in his practice and surrounding areas (see chapters 2 and 10). These are classically and beautifully expressed in his James Mackenzie 1978 lecture to the Royal College of General Practitioners. Needless to say, poor food quality is at the root of them. The McCarrison Society has been fortunate to have had the benefit of his nutritional wisdom as President for a number of years.

Dr E.F. Schumacher

Illustrative of the many disciplines with contributions to make to the ecology of health is the life and thought of Ernst Schumacher. Rhodes scholar, economist, author, farmer, journalist and academic, he brought his abilities to bear with great effect in the office of President of the Soil Association until his untimely death. One of his best-known contributions to the greater ecology is of course *Small is Beautiful*.

Dr Miles H. Robinson

A far-seeing American who, in his capacity as Scientific Advisor to the Citizens For Health Information Inc., based in Maryland, was greatly responsible for putting over the health potential of Cleave's work on refinement, overconsumption and dietary fibre in America.

J. I. Rodale

This perceptive American, whom detractors once described as an unsuccessful playwright turned 'health nut', has helped to conform my impression that an intelligent layman with an unsolved health problem is more likely to be successful at looking sideways at clues and findings already made, than the doctors themselves who make them.

Doctors have been well served for years with abstracts from the world of medicine, but with little or nothing from the world of health. Over the post-war years I have found Rodale's publication *Prevention* of tremendous help in reporting researchers into nutritional deficiencies. He brought to public attention some of the very earliest suspicions of the consequences of trace element deficiencies. His mantle has been ably continued by his son Robert. A fitting tribute to the house of Rodale was the publication by Rodale Press of the *Sunday Times Book of Real Bread*.

☆   ☆   ☆

The tongue of the wise is health.

Proverbs 12:18

REFERENCE

T.R. Allinson, *The Advantage of Wholemeal Bread* (London 1885).

Sir Albert Howard, *An Agricultural Testament* (OUP 1940).

Sir Albert Howard, *Farming and Gardening for Health or Disease* (Faber 1945).

R. McCarrison, *Nutrition and Health* (Faber 1953).

H.M. Sinclair, *The Work of Sir Robert McCarrison* (Faber 1953).

Weston Price, *Nutrition and Physical Degeneration* (American Academy of Applied Nutrition 1945).

Max O. Bircher-Benner, *Children's Diet* (C.W. Daniel Co. Ltd translated 1946).

T.L. Cleave, *The Saccharine Disease* (Wright 1974).

Brian Kellock, *The Fibre Man—Denis Burkitt* (Lion 1985).

Doris Grant, *Your Daily Food* (Faber 1973).

W.E. Tanner, *Arbuthnot Lane, His Life and Work* (Balliére Tyndal & Cox 1946).

Arbuthnot Lane, 'Preventable Disease Campaign' (*Daily Mail* Dec 29th 1925).

Everard Turner, 'Hygeia and Hippocrates' (*British Dental Journal* Oct 16th 1951).

W.E. Shewell-Cooper, *Soil Humus and Health* (Granada 1978).

Neil Painter, *Diverticular Disease of the Colon* (Heinemann 1975).

Avery Jones, *The Emergence of Gastro-Enterology* (Harveian Oration 1980).

Lionel Picton, *Thoughts on Feeding* (Faber 1946).

Eve Balfour, *The Living Soil* (Faber 1943).

Innes Pearse, *The Peckham Experiment* (Allen & Unwin 1943).

Kenneth Heaton, *Dietary Fibre* (Newman Publishing 1978).

Walter Yellowlees, 'Ill fares the land' (*Journal of the Royal College of General Practitioners* Jan 1979).

E.F. Schumacher, *Small is Beautiful* (Sphere Books Ltd 1973).

13
Political Priorities for Public Policies

The treatment of earth by man, the exploiter, is not only un-provident but sacrilegious. We are not likely to correct our hideous mistakes in this realm unless we can recover the mystical sense of oneness with Nature. I labour this precisely because many people think it fantastic; I think it fundamental to sanity.

William Temple
(Archbishop of Canterbury 1942-45).

A case has been made that simple purposeful changes in day-to-day living habits can reap great rewards in the betterment of personal health.

Any such benefits, especially in the longer term, can either be enhanced or negated by international, national and local community action or default. There is a desperate need for concerted action in the betterment of the environment.

International objectives

Few will grudge priority of attention given to those Third World countries in the starvation belts. Alongside their problems, ours of deplete food—and an excess of it at that—fall into perspective. Our patience in seeking to love our neighbours as ourselves may well be sorely tried as we become aware that tragic situations may be perpetuated or made worse by the political dogmatism of some native governments.

Clearly, and it is elemental truth, gifts of food and money

179

are at best first aid. Our best international efforts must be
along the lines of sharing the world's resources of energy,
development of water supplies, farming practice, conservation of organic matter, reforestation and the development of
local community health services.

The demand for and use of available energy

There is no more potent influence upon the health and disease
of the face of the earth and the life it supports than man's
inexorable demands for energy. Some two-thirds of the
world's population eke out meagre earth-surface fuel for the
sheer necessity of heat, light and survival. The remaining one-
third—which includes the West—is extravagant and wasteful
of energy in varying degrees. Bound up in the issue of the use
of fuel is that of the understandable desire of the individual to
be free to travel locally or worldwide in powered vehicles for
any purpose. Nevertheless, we have to face the fact that the
collective freedom of millions of individuals to travel millions
of miles daily by air or on land, has a tremendous impact on
our energy resources and upon pollution of the atmosphere.
How much longer before we are driven by fuel shortage, pollution and road congestion to define inessential journeys and
seek by education to achieve voluntary restriction? Should we
be prepared to fight to the death to defend a man's freedom to
jump into his car to go to the local shop when he runs out of
cigarettes? There is no doubt what health education should be
saying!

Through much of recorded history, life for the majority on
the planet has involved the endurance of uncomfortable heat
or cold, with cold predominating. Harsh cold winters of near
starvation were the norm for the majority until little more
than a hundred years ago; and that is how it is for much of the
Third World today—interspersed with periods of exhausting,
thirst-provoking heat.

To quote just one uncomfortable fact, a recent report of the
World Health Organisation states that about one half of the

world's women cook their families' meals on fires of wood, agricultural waste or dung—often inside small, poorly-ventilated huts—with appalling consequences to health. They would survive far longer inside a nuclear power station! We know, too, that they may have had to trek miles to find that ever more elusive wood which is disappearing faster than it is being replaced; all contributing to the march of the desert and near-perpetual drought. Even in the West, very many people find six to eight months of the year cold and miserable. The severity of winter conditions within the large land masses, such as the Soviet Union, is unenviable. As populations grow, the problem of keeping warm gets ever more expensive.

With the tilt of the earth's axis, our one sun does amazingly well for us over the greater part of the globe, but there is reason to believe it did even better for warmth under alternative geophysical conditions in time past. The visible evidence of coal and oil worldwide—including polar regions—suggests vastly more prolific conditions of growth than are obtained today. If we consider the volume of compressed vegetation represented in a seam of coal, it is impossible to conceive of today's annual scanty vegetation ever being a source of coal or oil. It is therefore tempting to consider the kind of conditions which could give rise to such profusion of growth worldwide.

Genesis speaks of a firmament, with waters above and waters below. (A marginal note refers to vapour above and waters below.) The concept of a time when the earth was substantially enveloped with water vapour is not new. The consequence of such would be a 'greenhouse effect' promoting luxuriant vegetation over the whole of the globe. The eventual descent of this mass of water in one or more deluges, precipitated by cataclysmic planetary events, is adequate to account for floods of global proportions, as in the time of Noah. Certainly, surveys of the ocean beds suggest a time when the sea level was very much lower than now.

These reflections are mentioned to suggest that by far and away the greatest untapped energy resource is the sun. If the sun exists just to sustain life on one of its planets the wastage of radiant heat into outer space is prodigious. And of even that tiny fraction which falls for the most part obliquely on the earth's surface the greater part is wasted.

Continuing research into the tapping of solar energy is therefore a must. Likewise every reasonable development of wind, wave, river and tidal power merits government encouragement. No other significant new source of energy seems likely to materialize in the near future, unless Professor Thomas Gold is right in prospecting vast quantities of methane deep beneath the earth's crust. Tantalizingly elusive is the prospect, one day, of separating off on a large scale the atoms of hydrogen and oxygen which comprise water, thereby unleashing two very active elements.

Nuclear energy

It is therefore necessary most carefully to consider the continuation and development of nuclear power if we are not to be faced with a very uncomfortable energy gap before the end of the century.

In so considering, I trust that my thinking revealed in this book is at least indicative of a lifelong concern regarding manmade and preventable hazards to health. I cannot discover any reason why I might have a blindspot in favour of nuclear energy or would support its potential unless I felt truly satisfied with its safety in relation to other sources of energy, which I do. I am entirely satisfied that British practice in regard to nuclear energy is able to produce large quantities of required energy with a health and safety potential for operatives and the public, far better than the comparable alternatives of coal, oil and gas.

The hazards of the latter fossil fuels include death and disability arising from mining, drilling, diving, traffic distribution hazards, risks of explosion and atmospheric pollution.

I can see no possible reason for Britain to modify its programme for nuclear energy given the types of reactor in use and safety and inspection standards, and the keeping of the opportunity for human error to an irreduceable minimum. Remembering the alarming accident in Chernobyl, in the Soviet Union, we must say that clearly the potential for safety of this type of reactor is not good. Also we are surrounded in Europe by other types of reactor. Very hard lessons have been learned. Nations will at all costs seek to avoid the international obloquy incurred by Chernobyl, although there may be hazards to be faced during the phasing out of these Leningrad-type reactors.

Nevertheless, public concern about nuclear energy is understandable and the invisibility of the hazard also lends itself to political mischief by those whose major target is nuclear weapons for defence. Radiation is inexorably linked in the public mind with one of man's most dreaded diseases—cancer—in regard to both cause and cure.

Governments will need to sustain vigorous campaigns of public reassurance if necessary programmes are to be maintained.

Hazards in perspective—the worst of all epidemics

Much of the measure of concern exhibited by modern man is related to the newsworthiness of the hazard. Nuclear energy is news; typhoid and legionnaires' disease, when they occur, are news; a plane crash is news. Yet the biggest single cause of premature death, certainly in Western society, continues to ravage almost unheeded.

I refer to the never-ending epidemic of so-called accidents in our midst. With accidents on the road, in the home and at work predominating.

I include this peril to health and safety because in addition to individual concern there is a tremendous responsibility devolving upon local and national governments. The fact is that the greater part of the millions of annual casualties in Britain alone are preventable.

To cause death or disablement by wilful carelessness is inexcusable. Unheeding self-injury is scarcely better. There are millions who must bear conscious or subconscious guilt and grief as a result of accidents which would be more fittingly described as 'avoidable bodily harm'. So many accidents result from inattention, laziness, arrogant overconfidence or being under the influence of drugs or alcohol.

There is considerable biblical reference to accidents and their prevention. As with disease, accidents are not visited upon man by the Lord. They arise from the exercise of our free will in the ordering of our daily lives. There is, however, much encouragement given to Christians in the matter of praying regularly for the safety of ourselves and loved ones as we come and go in the hazards of crowded living.

Conservation

Much that is put forward in this chapter, and the book as a whole, falls within the province of what in recent years has come to be known as conservation. Pre-eminent is the nurture of the land. Here I make a plea with every landowner and land manager to consider and conserve the precious inches of topsoil, the trees, the hedgerows and the wildlife. Our very health now and that of future generations depends upon this.

I urge that more of the great landowners follow the splendid example of parts of the Duchy of Cornwall estates in moving towards organic farming. The example could also be followed by the local authorities and public corporations who own farms.

I urge upon colleges of agriculture, worldwide, to ensure that the principles of organic agriculture are at least taught and demonstrated alongside the orthodox. I pray that policies be devised to encourage farmers to hold back from thrashing the land relentlessly, year after year, with machinery and maximum fertilizer application to produce crops of impoverished nutritional value far in excess of perceived need.

The population, food and resource equation

I will refrain from causing offence to some by pontificating about tackling the world's desperate population problem. But it needs to be said that if we are to feed ourselves and avoid diminishing the integrity of food, and if we are to help others to feed themselves, we must work with nature. Whatever mineral fertilizers we may deem necessary, we must at the same time ensure that all organic waste matter the world over is given opportunity, in the short or longer term, to be broken down by natural process and returned to the land. The burning of organic material must be a rare exception; municipal composting of carbonaceous household waste with the nitrogenous wastes of sewage must be an increasing priority. As of now, the chemical wastes of industry—particularly mercury, cadmium and lead—must be separately dealt with and kept free from municipal compost, rivers and sea.

The issue over fertilizers and pesticides has been discussed in chapter 3. The point to be made now is that the monitoring and control of these matters must be a continuing priority of the World Health Organisation, the Food and Agriculture Organisation, and the government of every nation. There could have been no grimmer or more urgent warning to the world of the lethal potential of the basic ingredients of agricultural pesticides than the Bhopal disaster in 1984. Deadly methyl isocyanate gas was inhaled by a quarter of a million Indians, killing 2,500 people—the greatest industrial disaster of all time.

Rainfall and water

Crucial to the practice of conservation and to health is water supply. Climate changes which are at least partly caused by man, are making it increasingly difficult to ensure that available rainwater matches the demands of the populations. There has been serious deficiency in some recent years, even in the usually wet westlands of Britain. Further south, around the Mediterranean, shortages have been so acute that inhabitants have been endeavouring to turn away holidaymakers. Other parts of the world have been getting too much water.

For years now, in Britain, recycling water has been necessary. In the case of the River Thames for instance—which receives the treated effluents from numerous sewage plants and from which public water supply is drawn at intervening points—recycling necessarily takes place several times over from source to mouth. Inherent in the purification process is the use of significant amounts of chlorine each time round. Chlorine deals effectively with the bacteria which can be seen under basic microscopes, but there is increasing doubt as to its effectiveness against the proliferating variety of mini-viruses, and concern that their survival accounts for much of the endemic 'tummy' upsets, for which no satisfactory cause is found. Recycled water must also inevitably carry a build-up of excreted drug and hormone residues. Having mentioned the Thames I hasten to add that the authority responsible for London's water is one of the most efficient in the world.

Nitrates and fluorides

Our representatives need also to be vigilant about the levels of nitrates in our water supplies. Many experts consider that present levels are unacceptable—the formation of carcinogens being of particular concern. Reference must also be made to fluorine. There is a debate as to whether or not this is an essential trace element. On balance, I believe it is. If it is, the normal and natural source should be through our food, but there is very little present in deplete food. Its source would certainly not normally be our water supply. Its presence in a few waters is incidental. In my opinion, the addition of unnatural complex fluoride to water supplies for the sake of children's teeth is an unacceptable method of attempting to achieve a trace of fluorine into our intricate biological systems.

Thinking the unthinkable—a thought for the future

The 'unthinkable' is now to pose the question: is the flush toilet water-carriage system, whose introduction a century ago was life-saving against typhoid fever, cholera, dysentery and the like, now outdated and unsuited to twenty-first-century living? Does it make sense to use some 40% of precious domestic water supply to flush the body's germ-laden waste into our water-supplying rivers or into the increasingly polluted sea? Does it make sense to lose incessantly these vast quantities of our land's fertility? Would the teeming millions of China be so self-sufficient in food had all their wastes been directed into water-carriage systems?

We may be forced to do some radical rethinking. In the meantime I would certainly advise any rural dweller faced with the decision and expense of sewer connection to consider the modern alternatives of local reintegration of waste through microbial activity, all very much within the principles of conservation and using methods now vastly superior to the old cesspools and septic tanks.

The tree and the forest

Intimately linked with rainfall are the trees on the face of the earth. Crucial to life itself as Moses reminds us ('The tree of the field is man's life'). There can be no doubt that man's hunger for wood worldwide has had significant effect on climate and rainfall.

Trees are indeed a precious resource provided in abundance for man from his earliest days on earth, but he has continued to reduce their number ever since. This was tolerable when the world population was small. Today's population explosion and its demand upon the tree and its products is removing the remaining trees at a terrifying rate. And it is not only industrialized man who is doing it! At least two-thirds of the word's population is reliant upon wood for warmth and cooking. Many people walk miles each day for supplies, stripping the forests and pushing forward desert borders. Long gone are the biblical forests, the cedars of Lebanon, the forests of Arabia, the vineyards, olive yards and fruit trees of Canaan, and much of the great forests of Africa, America, Europe and the Soviet Union.

This relentless deforestation is more than enough to account for some of the dramatic and continuing changes in the world's rainfall and desertification. We must tackle reforestation as a matter of worldwide urgency. Few countries are taking this seriously. Those who try, like Britain, are tending to replace former rich broadleaf woodland with clone-like conifers, which are a drain upon, rather than an improver of the forest floor.

However much fossil fuels need to be conserved, advanced nations must be prepared to reduce the use of wood, even being willing to ship it in redundant tankers to the Third World to tide them over, while reforestation proceeds. Advanced nations using dwindling earth surface resources for fuel, or making fuel, is now inexcusable. The trendy wood-burning stoves of the West, and our extravagant use of paper, are indulgences we cannot continue much longer. The burning of dung for fuel in the Third World is no less regrettable, as it robs the land of precious fertility, but without our long-term help many have little option but to continue these self-defeating practices.

Prototype for the future?

There is a township, perhaps the only one, where by voluntary consent the inhabitants continue to live within the spirit of conservation. The place is Davis, near Sacramento, USA. There, by dint of an active co-operation between the micicipality, a small university and an agricultural college, an ecological way of life is practised, having maximum concern for natural resources. The growth of the town is constrained. All new properties are sited and equipped to make maximum use of solar energy. Older properties are required to comply on changing hands. The demands on other forms of energy are dramatically reduced. All possible organic waste is recycled. We look forward to hearing more of their experience and results.

It is an objective of this book to encourage healthier ways of living for the individual, the family and the community. Increasingly a silent majority can see the wisdom of many of the precepts of the conservation lobby, but are put off by the antics and lifestyle of some of the more extreme proponents.

We already know enough to be building into our environment the blueprint for the future. Is it too much to hope that the current surge of interest and awakening of the public in matters of health and the environment will attract in common cause leaders of discernment from the community and all political parties?

This is not merely an aspiration for Britain, or Europe, or the West. It is a worldwide challenge to mankind to rescue the living face of the earth from mounting depletion and pollution.

The resources of the earth should be used as God's gifts to the whole human race and used with due consideration for the needs of the present and future generations.

Resolution at Malvern Conference of Christian churches (1945)

14
Health and the Christian

Christians are liable to the same lack of awareness, indifference and ignorance of the precepts of health as non-Christians. Some Christians shy away from the conscious effort necessary to walk the path of health, as pandering to the flesh. To such I maintain that the building up and preservation of personal health, and that of others in our charge, is a Christian duty and a worthy objective for all mankind.

Mark and Ruth are not untypical of conscientious parents we have known, who gave of themselves freely to the work of the church, especially with young people. Yet, time and time again, their efforts were dogged by the family's obvious ill-health. They never complained but clearly, at times, the extra effort of their Christian work, added to all their home responsibilities on a very modest salary, appeared to push them to the limit of their strength.

We were asked to have a quiet word with them at a time when they were extremely low with family illness. They were very touched by their friends' concern about their poor health, but clearly it never occurred to them that there might be anything in their lifestyles to account for it. 'After all, our doctor has never mentioned this possibility . . . our health is surely in the hands of the Lord,' they mused. 'He knows our problems and we look to him for the strength to overcome them. Some of our other Christian friends would almost certainly feel we would be selfish and wrong to divert already precious time from furthering the gospel to concern ourselves about whether or not our eating habits are at fault.'

'Do not worry'

At first thought, these unselfish sentiments might seem to be wholly in the spirit of that part of the Sermon on the Mount which enjoins man not to worry about his life, what he will eat or drink, or about his body (Matthew 6:25, NIV). But if we look at the whole context of this injunction, we see that our Lord's purpose was to establish priorities for his followers. Unlike the pagan, whose preoccupation was possessions, clothes, food and drink, the first priority of the Christian was to seek the kingdom of God who, in turn, would provide for all his daily needs.

The emphasis here is on not worrying or being anxious about food, drink and the body. This is a very different thing from exercising a wise and discerning choice from the profusion of foods on the supermarket shelf in order to feed life to our living tissues.

In verse 27, our Lord goes on to ask: 'Who of you by worrying can add a single hour to his life?' How very true! We have an inbuilt potential life-span and nothing we can do by any means can prolong it. But, there is a great deal we can do, by neglect, to shorten our span of life. Unwise and continuing poor choice of food is the surest way of knocking years off our life's potential.

The essence of the message we carry forward from the Sermon on the Mount is that, having grasped the principles of healthy living, their application falls into perspective in their routine daily living. Nothing advised in this book is intended to justify any kind of obsessional preoccupation with food or health.

I have found much encouragement over the years in the work and testimony of individual Christians in the interests of health, but little or no interest in the mainstream Protestant or Catholic churches in the health of their membership. Much more concern and Bible-based teaching has been manifest in the writings of the Seventh Day Adventists and even Jehovah's Witnesses, notwithstanding doctrinal differences in other matters of the Christian faith.

Some forty years ago the Salvation Army, encouraged by Christian doctors, was already setting a fine example in healthy wholefood feeding in some of their children's homes. Even earlier, I encountered considerable food enlightenment in some of the wartime canteens of the Mission to Mediterranean Garrisons. This contrasts starkly with lifeless food since met with at various Christian conference centres, and even at some harvest suppers!

I have also scanned the bookshelves over the years hoping that Christian writers might see the relevance of physical health to the promotion of spiritual health. Either such books were not written or I did not find them. What I did find was an immense amount of writing about being healed from states of sickness and disease.

There was endless speculation as to whether or not God, as part of his pruning process, visited sickness upon us. And why did he permit the cruelty of disease? Did Satan cause disease? Why was healing in response to prayer, even in the absence of faith on the part of the patient, sometimes accomplished rapidly and decisively? And why was healing sometimes not manifest in the cases of some of the most God-fearing, including ministers of the gospel, with many praying fervently on their behalf?

It seems that just as in the world of medicine, the spiritual realms of cure and healing are found to be much more interesting than merely staying in health.

God cares about our health

It is only lately, when I was well advanced in drafting these pages, that I found what I had been looking for, for so long. And then I didn't find it—it found me! I was sent a copy of *God Wants You Whole* by Selwyn Hughes. What a thrill, at last, to find a great evangelist and Bible scholar affirming that God cares passionately about our state of health on earth, and that Christ laid down his life not only for the spiritual ills of mankind but for their physical sicknesses as well. The book provides wise, scripturally sound and purposeful advice—including the wise choice of food—for staying in health. One can only add, 'Amen!'

I was particularly taken with the conclusions of his painstaking research into the real meaning of suffering which he shows in biblical context. It has much more to do with spiritual affliction than bearing or carrying a sickness. Hughes contends—and I profoundly agree—that suffering we accept; sickness we resist. He reminds us that Jesus proclaimed no beatitude for sickness. There is nothing blessed about it! Indeed, nowhere does Jesus say that it is blessed to be physically or mentally afflicted, blind, crippled, in pain or diseased. On the contrary, in such conditions, he was moved with compassion and when asked, invariably healed.

God does not bring illness and disease

It could well be comforting and encouraging to many who are burdened with grievous and prolonged illness to be assured that it is no part of God's pruning or chastening purpose to visit or inflict illness or disease upon us. When disease does arise, he can and does use it, as he can use all circumstances, for our spiritual growth, which includes giving us the strength to bear the affliction. But the very realization that God did not bring the illness, and would rather that we had never got it, and does not want us to go on enduring it if we can be healed, must surely assist healing and relief. This is a long way from the teaching of passive acceptance prevalent among Christians well into the twentieth century.

I am not unmindful of the large number of people very severely physically or mentally handicapped. Healing and restoration for such may only, at best, be partial and even then forged upon the efforts of long patient rehabilitation.

Health is loving our neighbour

If I may presume yet again to discern the Lord's will in this matter, I believe he pleads with man to conduct himself, to love his neighbour and to live with and use the resources of the earth in such a way that disease and disability are prevented with all the knowledge and means at his disposal. This involves searching reappraisal of almost every facet of our way of life. Sexual behaviour at variance with God's law and the millions of innocent victims down the ages; exploitation of the fertility of the earth for excess profit, and the consequences of resultant famine and depletion; mindless attitudes to road safety and the millions of victims . . . and much, much more. May we always be ready, graciously to contend with those who would blame God. The fact is that God has given us this world and we can make what we will of it (Psalm 115:16). Our help in this is his word, divine guidance and the Holy Spirit.

It is a sad mistake to assume that God is only interested in our spiritual life and immortal being. On the contrary, Paul emphasizes in Romans 8:11 that the great power of the same Holy Spirit which raised up Jesus from the dead is freely available to quicken our mortal bodies. Again, Paul affirms the Lord's interest in the preservation of our whole spirit and soul and body (1 Thessalonians 5:23).

Christians can readily accept that God, by the provision and sacrifice of his only Son our Lord Jesus Christ, the gift of the Holy Spirit and the Scriptures, has provided all things necessary for the promotion and maintenance of the spiritual life of his children. What Christians have so often failed to recognize is that, given an earthly and physical dispensation as a foundation to eternal life, God likewise provided all things necessary to the promotion and maintenance of physical health. This he did by the bountiful provision of the fruits of the earth and the soil from which all living creatures stem.

The Lord, through his scribes, set down in the Scriptures his commandments for our spiritual guidance. Likewise, he set down his blueprint for our physical use of planet earth, its resources and management.

Down through the ages, disobedience to God and rejection of the saving grace of our Lord Jesus Christ, has had manifestly appalling consequences for mankind. Similarly—and indeed as part of the same—rejection and disregard of divine guidance in the matter of our physical health has been a tragedy for all mankind and particularly for Christians who have the means to know better.

The body, the temple of the Holy Spirit

Very pertinently indeed, Paul advises us that the body is the temple of the indwelling Holy Spirit and it behoves us to keep it in good shape (1 Corinthians 3:16-17).

There are very few Christians who, when illness strikes, are not prepared to resort to medical help—and rightly so. It may take weeks, months or years to get them fit again and while the illness prevails, it is a hindrance to work of any kind, including the Lord's work. Yet some of these same Christians, when not in sickness, feel inhibited about devoting a fraction of such time to the adoption of healthy routine habits of daily living. They somehow feel that it is a spiritually unprofitable fleshly diversion.

If anything I am saying opens up the smallest glimmer of new light, I do urge you to supplement it by reading *God Wants You Whole*.

The Lord God has provided a wondrous creation of infinite variety. He has endowed nature as an open book to be read. He has gifted man with powers of observation and deduction. From the time that man first planted seeds in the ground God has enabled him to learn the conditions best favouring growth. He ensured that man would learn that if he means to go on sowing seeds in the same ground he must return the wastes of nature to it. He knew that man would discover that if he did not, he would get poor and diseased crops.

The Lord God knew that man could easily discover that the

health or disease of his livestock was closely related to the health of the plants and herbs upon which they fed.

The Lord God would credit man by simple observation to relate the quality of his own health with that of the plants, seeds, herbs and meat he took for food. Countless humble men of the soil down through the ages have learned these lessons and passed them on to their sons and daughters. Yet it is astonishing that scientific man can have reached such an advanced state of twentieth-century knowledge without having grasped the ecological message of soil, food and health.

Crucial to man's understanding of God's bountiful provision for his earthly needs is an adequate knowledge of all that the Old Testament has to say about it, including the law. Christians rightly appreciate that they are released from the burden of the law through redemption by our Lord Jesus Christ. Many—particularly young Christians in claiming the provision of grace—now feel that the Old Testament has little to offer in the Christian life. They make a sad mistake in passing over the wealth of wisdom which the law provides.

☆   ☆   ☆

Your statutes are wonderful; therefore I obey them. The entrance of your words gives light; it gives understanding to the simple.

Psalm 119:129-130, NIV.

From John Byrom, author of 'Christians Awake' to his wife in Salford England.

Trinity College Cambridge, Sat Dec 7th, 1729

My dear love,
    . . . I am sure that herbs, roots and fruits in season, good house bread, water porridge, fresh milk and the like are the properest food for the children. Puddings and dumplings are a

sort of bread and so may be very good for 'em if the meal or flour be so; but to take bread and crumble it and sugar it and plum it and boil it, is to take much pains to turn wholesome nourishment into unwholesome, as if that which disguises it from natural taste, the sugar and sweets were away it would soon be rejected as having lost all its proper nourishing sweetness, as much as green gooseberries, apricots and the like would be rejected as not having yet got their nourishing sweetness if they were not buried in sugar.

. . . Good night my love,

John

(Extract from personal communication from the Medical Officer of Health Salford, 1956. This great Christian scholar John Byrom also studied medicine in France for several years and was called by his friends 'the doctor'.)

REFERENCE

A.B. Cunning, F.R. Innes, *We Are What We Eat* (Salvationist Publishing 1954).

Selwyn Hughes, *God Wants You Whole* (Kingsway Publications 1984).

15
Journey into Health and Life

This rather personal chapter is included in the hope that it may be of help to others who are on the journey into life, but like me may not realize it until it draws to a close.

There are many who can testify to having been guided and sustained by the hand of the Lord on life's journey and who will say that, having grasped his hand in faith, he never let them down. It is a common experience that the way can be rough and perplexing. It may seem impossible to see any purpose in some of the trials and tribulations or diversions at the time.

Perhaps one of the greatest joys accorded to those Christians who survive to maturity is to be able to see a purpose and fitting together of events which had previously seemed totally inexplicable.

It has been said that one of the greatest purposes of biblical prophecy is to appreciate, in retrospect, how beautifully and faithfully all the great sequence of prophecies is being fulfilled —a tremendous fillip to the faith of Christians! It is also a great uplift to personal faith to begin to see, with hindsight, a purpose in the working out of events in our own lives, the lives of our forefathers and the lives of others. But there are some cautionary notes to be sounded! The first is to be aware of the pitfall of spiritual arrogance: to assume that we have achieved anything worth while in life other than satisfying ambition and ego; to dare to presume that we may have been used by God for any purpose, or to seek to use God to justify our ideas. Secondly, we must seek to avoid the well-known liability to see past events through rose-coloured spectacles. Finally, we must avoid overindulgence in the past in favour of looking forward and looking up.

Subject to all of these, I can only declare that over many years I have become increasingly conscious that the Lord cares deeply about the health of the earth, its vegetation and wildlife, and of his human kind. I am not alone in such consciousness—non-Christians also can be very diligent in the preservation of the living environment.

For my part, I cannot escape the conclusion that notwithstanding volition and in spite of (or even because of) early events in life, some of the places I have been caused to visit, people I have been privileged to meet and the work of others I have been caused to digest must have a meaning beyond co-incidence.

By way of illustration of a likely purpose in an unwanted circumstance, I cite a frustrating handicap which came upon me round about the age of eleven. I became extremely short sighted, necessitating the wearing of the very unsightly spectacles of that time. I was progressively rendered more useless at ball games, and felt very 'out of things' in my teens at the very sport-orientated Plymouth College. I did not think very much of myself at that time.

I railed against the God of my parents for lumbering me with this handicap and it was my excuse for teenage rebellion against anything to do with religion. The scientific materialism of Medical School pushed God even further away, and it was not to be until I was in my early twenties that I was constrained to call upon him. It was following a night-long wartime blitz in my London teaching hospital. The city about was already devastated, but as dawn broke we saw that miraculously St Paul's Cathedral had again survived. This had to be the hand of God. We were all very tired. Some of us had final qualifying examinations to be taken in a few hours' time. Before falling on my bed, I dropped to my knees and pleaded:

'God, you know what's been going on these past months. If I pass today it will be a miracle of your doing, and I will never cease to be grateful.' God saw me through but it was to be at least a further three years before I fully acknowledged him, as was his due. We so easily hold back on our promises to God. I can appreciate now the value of faithful and praying parents, god-parents and friends. It is so important that we, in turn, remember to pray for those in our charge.

In the meantime—and I take no credit—it has come to pass that the greater part of my life has been orientated towards preventive medicine and to exhortation of a reluctant community towards healthier ways of living, with an emphasis on the integrity of the daily food.

Towards the close of a professional lifetime, I can now see that my erstwhile hated short sight played no small part in my journey and arrival at this point. Even as a schoolboy, and later as a medical student, I explored everything there was to be read about short sight and its possible causes. The only inferences to be gleaned were a hereditary tendency and the possibility of a nurtural cause of deficiency of vital nutrients during the period of rapid childhood growth. Thus was the seed of nutritional interest first implanted. The fact of short sight was again critical in the matter of war service. It ensured that, as an Army Medical Officer, I served away from active combat and in some places of fascinating interest, culminating with the privilege of several years in unforgettable Jerusalem.

Cradle of health

During a journey of several thousands of miles through Algeria, Tunisia, Egypt, Sinai and the Gaza Strip on route to Palestine, the revelation of health began to dawn on me. For most of that journey the land was dead and lifeless, unless a natural water supply encouraged cultivation. The nomadic natives seemed to do little more than scratch the surface. At the end of the journey in the hinterland of Jaffa suddenly there was lush vegetation—orange groves, fruit, cereals and vegetables, not due to natural resources, but to a sturdy, enterprising people at work. They were Jewish immigrants (later to be increased in numbers by refugees from the European holocaust). They were of healthy appearance, especially the beautiful children of the kibbutzim, contrasting starkly with the tragically undernourished and fly-infested children along the desert way. The clear inference was that the health of a people is directly proportional to the nurture and fertility of the land and the sense of purpose of its inhabitants. The steady 'plop-plop' of pumping engines signified a constant flow of life-giving water. Later, part of Palestine was declared the new State of Israel.

They were again beginning to inhabit 'a land I [the Lord] had searched out for them . . . the most beautiful of all lands' (Ezekiel 20:6, NIV).

Spiritual rejuvenation

Exploring Palestine from Gaza to Galilee, one became increasingly gripped with the certainty that these were the very places where our Lord had walked and prayed, and the literal truth of the gospels was compelling.

One does not have to visit the Holy Land to experience spiritual renewal, but to be given the privilege of sojourning there, and then failing to be touched by the Spirit of the living Lord, would be blindness indeed. I could see that many of my friends and colleagues were similarly moved.

It was during my third year in Palestine that I was to meet Nancy—the love of my life—an Army Nursing Sister. And what more unforgettable place to meet than on the Mount of Olives! She was only briefly in Palestine by what seemed the remotest chance, having been diverted from a journey which would have otherwise taken her three thousand miles away. We explored together the city of the great King, walked the Judean hills, Carmel, Jericho and the Dead Sea. Within the space of a few months we were married in Jerusalem Cathedral.

The long weary war was drawing to a close, and even the

'powers that be' were helpful in not posting us to be more than a hundred miles apart! After a year of 'brief encounters' and heart-tugging separations, we were able to sail home together on a P&O troopship.

We would not have missed that further year in Palestine as it afforded us the exceptional spiritual experience of the fellowship we shared with the Shelley/Campion family—both in Jerusalem and Cyprus. Edgar Shelley, who will be known to hundreds of servicemen and women, was Life President of the Jerusalem Chamber of Commerce and he and his wife, Blanche, were tremendous 'on-the-spot' teachers of Second Advent truths. It was an unforgettable experience to share in the breaking of bread in the upper room of their house overlooking the Old City and Mount Zion. They taught the history and purpose of the Israeli people and we learned one of life's most important lessons for Christians—to repent of the blind, cruel and hypocritical treatment of the Jews down the ages, to befriend them and share the gospel, for they continue to be 'the apple of the Lord's eye'. To the Jews we owe the receiving, recording and working out of the Mosaic law, so crucial to our understanding of hygiene and a healthful moral code. Through their Passover, their trials, their testing and suffering, they made the way possible for Christians to find their passover—which is Christ Jesus. From the Shelleys, we discovered the incredible relevance to daily events by reading together *Daily Light*.

There was also the opportunity for further fellowship with the unforgettable Joe Fison—the Army Chaplain who married us—a fire for God, destined to become a senior bishop.

Back in post-war Britain there were all the understandable inclinations to take immediate employment. However, I shall always be grateful for the nudgings and promptings which caused me instead to set aside a couple of precious years to qualify in Public Health and, even more so, again with help from on high, to proceed to a Doctorate in my university. This was to prove of inestimable help in being listened to in the unpopular and unglamorous corridors of preventive medicine.

Meanwhile, Nancy and I continued to meet with very special people in our professional and spiritual life, including a number of those of our generation named as Apostles of Health in chapter 12.

There is one further subject which I feel sure the Lord has wished to bring to my attention in the context of prevention. I refer to the consequences of modern medical treatment and technology upon the process of dying when life's span has run its course.

Eastbourne, and the whole of the south coast of England, has one of the highest concentrations of elderly people in the world. I was responsible for a wide range of community services for their care. I had opportunity to see at first hand many of the hazards which befall the aged sick and their relatives and helpers.

I was invited to address a large international health congress, meeting in Eastbourne, on the subject of the hazards of old age. I prepared my paper and slides very carefully, making mention of the part doctors and nurses can so easily and unwittingly play in the powerful and undignified prolongation of life of the aged sick by modern intensive therapy. It was a good session, with questions and discussion and no hint of misunderstanding. However, within hours, sections of the press chose to confuse the issue of medicated survival with that of positive euthanasia . . . in spite of the fact that I spoke explicitly against the latter! The furore of press, radio and television was unpleasant while it lasted, but I felt throughout it all that the Lord had this situation firmly in control, and the counter-reaction that followed within a week was heartwarming as hundreds of letters, from all over the world, came to me from folk who were suffering undignified and painful prolongation of life, and from friends and relatives of many more.

It had all been worth while to have received this sad but wonderful dossier of case histories. I was later given encouraging opportunity to enlarge upon the subject and write further—particularly in America where there is great understanding in the matter. The experience has been invaluable to

me in contributing professionally to helping with the foundation of a Christian hospice.

A philosophy of health and life

We are blessed with four lovely children and are grateful to
them for being unwitting subjects in our working out the essentials of health and life in a challenging world. We thank
them, and are now deeply touched that, in varying emphasis
and degree, they and their partners have carried these forward into their own homes and careers and that we see further
fulfilment in our grand-children.

As we draw to a conclusion we are thus encouraged by our
family to feel able to use a collective 'we' in these writings. We
would like to feel that if only a few of the understandings
which have come to us and helped us along the way are of help
to others, writing them down will have been worth while.
While we have no hesitation in commending our overall concept of positive health, it would be too much to expect readers
to agree with all our suggestions. In the matter of health—as
in all things—it is essential to see the wood for the trees!

Ideally, in our vision, the health-seeking individual and
family will be confident that health is a personal and family
responsibility and that a great part of its attainment is in our
own hands. The pursuit of health will be relaxed and part and
parcel of a normal way of life. It will be followed without
anxiety and too much preoccupation over detail. It will include concern over the safe-keeping of the environment and
the husbanding and recycling of precious resources.

Illness can and does occur, even where the daily living is
conscientious. We must not be dismayed or fearsome. We
must not lose confidence, even where such as inexplicable
congenital deformity occurs, or where occasionally the very
teachers of wholeness and health may die young.

We are deeply grateful to the Lord for leading us along
life's journey of absorbing interest and for our many totally
undeserved blessings, notwithstanding our waverings of faith,

backslidings and failures. Our conclusion is, as in the words of his servant of old: 'For we cannot but speak the things which we have seen and heard' (Acts 4:20). And we continue with the greatest of these in the concluding chapter.

☆   ☆   ☆

I will instruct you and teach you in the way you should go.
Psalm 32:8, NIV.

I am the way, the truth and the light.
John 14:6.

REFERENCE

Daily Light (Samuel Bagster).

Kenneth Vickery, 'The Hazards of Retirement' (*Royal Society of Health Journal* July 1969).

Kenneth Vickery, 'Medicated Survival, the Press—the Public—the Professions and the Patient' (Royal Society of Health 1974).

Kenneth Vickery, 'The Right to be Allowed to Die' (*This Week,* New York 1969).

F.W. Dillistone, *The Life Of Joe Fison—Afire for God* (Amate Press 1983).

16
Choose Life

It has been said that the truest end of life, is to know that life never ends. I prefer to modify this and say that 'life *need* never end'!

This present life tastes good to many and, judging by the endeavours of man to prolong it, is sweet and very precious. Choosing health is important to its best fulfilment and the attainment of our maximum expectation of life.

Yet we are constantly reminded—and very pointedly during funeral services—that 'man's days on earth are as a flower in the field, or a mist which appears for a while and then vanishes'. We are urged to pray to be taught to number our days that we may apply our hearts to wisdom.

Millions down the ages have declared that the greatest wisdom we can acquire during these few fleeting years, is to be provided with the opportunity and choice to break out of the time warp of a life span on earth into eternal life.

Choosing health can be a way, but by no means the only way, through which our eyes may be opened to responding to one of the most significant invitations given to man by God, which is 'choose life'. These very words are given to us in all major English translations in Deuteronomy 30:19 coupled with the alternative of choosing death. The prospects of either blessing or cursing are repeated throughout the Bible, culminating in the New Testament.

Life eternal

The life so commended is a life vastly more precious and enduring than this short earthly estate where the soul is briefly manifest in the dense matter of the present world. To have lived on earth is to have become eligible for the gift of eternal life which was from the beginning, and ever shall be. There is the offer of transforming this transitory life where we have glimpsed briefly, as through a glass darkly, the wonders of our God. It is the fulfilment of the most precious gift obtainable. It is the life of God revealed in Jesus Christ by his Holy Spirit. It is eternal because it was from the eternity which is past, is now, and which is to come.

Blood: essential for life temporal and eternal

In chapter 5 we saw some of the remarkable provisions for the health of man on earth embodied in the law given through Moses. We also touched upon some of the wonderful life-sustaining properties of blood. A large part of the same law dealt with animal sacrifice. This was the dispensation when God was working out the pre-Christian part of his plan for the redemption of man through his demonstration people, Israel. They were the subject of God's tremendous promises and covenants, all of which were honoured or are yet to be. The sacrificial animals were typified by the lamb and the sprinkling of blood was central to the ceremonial requirement. Even the Lord's chosen and particular people were wayward, stubborn, spiritually blind and sinful. These offerings were God's provision to cover and pass over their guilt, pending the fore-ordained, once and for ever sufficient sacrifice of our Lord Jesus Christ.

There are certain words of Scripture which are said to be off-putting to some Christians and would-be Christians—the blood is one of them. Yet it cannot be avoided if any consideration of health and life is to be effective.

So we remind ourselves of the pertinent relevance of the

familiar words in the Holy Communion Service: 'Lamb of God . . . that takes away the sins of the world,' and, 'The blood of our Lord Jesus Christ which was shed for you; preserve your body and soul into everlasting life.'

For everlasting life we need a blood transfusion. We require blood that is suitable, available and acceptable. Our Lord Jesus Christ is the Donor, the true universal Donor. His blood —in the emblem of the wine—is the strength of life, just as we have seen his body—in the emblem of the bread—is the sustenance of life.

There must be no misunderstanding in regard to the place of health. There is no pre-condition to eternal life apart from personal belief and repentance. Bodily health is vital to the wholeness of health in this earthly estate, but it is no requirement to the fullness of life eternal. Health is a worthy aspiration of man. It is commended here as a path by which man may better see the bountiful provision of God expressed in Scripture and in nature. With such wonders evident in this earthly estate, how much more we should be able to take his word of greater wonders beyond. For those who have found eternal life first, health is commended as a worthy supplementary discipline for the Christian, to enhance the maximum of bodily and spiritual vigour. Whichever way arrived at, health here and now is not whole nor complete unless it is embraced by the spiritual dimension. And the one and only spiritual dimension which is itself whole and complete is the Christian one.

We venture in reverence to see in the Godhead that same ecological principle which he manifests throughout nature of the parts working together in unity and wholeness: Father, Son and Holy Spirit.

Priorities

Our concept throughout has been that of health as physical, mental and spiritual. 'Surely,' it may be asked, 'is that not a wrong order of priority?' I leave Paul to answer that, and quote:

> If there is a natural body there is also a spiritual body . . . the first
> man Adam became a living being, the last Adam, a life-giving
> Spirit. The spiritual did not come first, but the natural, and after
> that the spiritual (1 Corinthians 15:44-46, NIV).

Nevertheless, that which comes last, as in the pages of this
book, is by far and away of greatest import!

The daily nourishment of the spiritual life is prayer. The
Christian requires no further commendation than that of his
Lord, that men ought always to pray. Man's motive in obeying
is not that of secondary benefit, but it is comforting to know
that prayer can be important to health.

Pray—it's healthy

. . . so read a *Daily Mail* headline, based on the experience of
a Dr Herbert Benson in America. Regular prayer, he claims,
is good for high blood pressure, anxiety and stress. The prescription of this Harvard physician is: 'Close the eyes, breathe
deeply and pray for twenty minutes twice a day.' His is by no
means the first such exhortation and helps add credibility to
the observation that though it may cost much to be a practising Christian it may, in fact, cost very much more—even in
this earthly state—not to be one!

. . . that seeing they might not see . . .

Just as in the matter of health, whose precepts are there to be
read in the book of nature, there is a remarkably similar blindness hindering man from grasping the stupendously more
precious gift of life to be read in the Book of Life. And, as in
the sciences, there are the 'monologists' who can only see part
of the whole.

But here the simile ends. Life eternal cannot be attained by
human effort. The hand of the Lord is held out to us, and is to
be grasped by faith and understanding of the promises of
God, such as the assurance in John 20:31:

These [signs] are written that you may believe that Jesus is the Christ, the Son of God, and that believing you may have life in his name (RSV).

Many are the books which have been written explaining further what is required of us by way of belief, faith and repentance in securing the gift of life. With their help we can have our eyes opened to the significance of the breath of life, the tree of life, the fountain of life, the promise of life, the book of life and the crown of life and, so relevant to our spiritual blindness, the pride of life.

But one book above all others, and the culmination of the whole Bible in the matter of life, is the Gospel of John. Attractive in its simple form, but even more compelling in the modern illustrated form, such as one of the inexpensive presentations by Creative Publishing—*The Offer of Life*.

If what has been said about the worthwhileness of health for even this transitory life makes a grain of sense, I plead with you to go forward in wholeness of body, mind and Spirit to claim the infinitely more wonderful and enduring gift of eternal life: 'He who has the Son has life; he who does not have the Son of God does not have life' (1 John 5: 12, NIV). Therefore, choose *life*!

'Now this is eternal life: that they may know you, the only true God, and Jesus Christ, whom you have sent' (John 17:3, NIV).

REFERENCE

The Offer of Life: The Gospel of John (Creative Publishing 1982, 1983).

Shaun Usher, 'Pray—It's Healthy' (*Daily Mail* March 30th 1979).

Glossary

Allergy A state of abnormal and individual hypersensitivity—the more normal response to the provoking substance being immunity.

Antibodies Substances in blood which neutralize bacterial toxins.

Anti-oxidants Substances which inhibit decomposition.

Carcinogens Substances causing or percipitating cancer.

Chemotherapy Treatment using chemical agents.

Cholesterol An essential substance derived from animal fats. Also manufactured in the body. Vital for nerve tissues, bile and fatty acids. Body can receive too much of it.

Clinical ecology Study of how the environment promotes health and disease.

Compost The result of any system of mixing and decaying natural wastes in a heap or pit in order to obtain a product resembling the leaf mould of the forest floor.

Coronary Related to the coronary vessels which supply blood to the heart. Commonly used to denote heart attack due to blockage.

Congenital Existing at birth.

Diabetes A breakdown of the body's sugar/insulin control.

Double-blind Refers to studies designed to reveal if drugs or other treatments produce statistically significant benefits. Patients, controls, doctors and assessors are kept uninformed of who gets what.

Enzyme A protein substance which facilitates biological reactions.

Epidemiology The distribution and relationship of diseases
with factors in the environment. Study hitherto largely confined to the infections. Now seen as a valuable tool for all
diseases.

Euthanasia An easy death. Connoted to imply the purposeful
hastening of death to relieve suffering.

Gamma rays High energy electromagnetic radiation, similar
to X-rays with considerable power of penetration.

Hormones Chemical compounds produced in one organ carried in blood and circulating fluids to stimulate activity elsewhere.

Ions Atoms, or groups of atoms, electrically charged. Very
significant in the functioning of the heart pacemaker and
nerve junctions in the brain.

Mutation Change in structure of the gene which carries the
blueprint for correct cell reproduction.

Organic Derived from living organisms. As applied to farming
denotes avoidance of artificial fertilizers and chemical
pesticides.

Pathogenic Capable of causing disease.

Psychotrophic Relating to drugs which affect mood.

Thrombosis Clotting of blood in vessels. Gravely encountered
in vessels of heart, brain, lungs and abdomen.

God Wants You Whole
The Way to Healing, Health and Wholeness

by Selwyn Hughes

If God is always willing to heal, why do people remain ill—even when they have faith for healing?

How can we all live more healthy lives, day by day?

With openness and honesty, Selwyn Hughes faces squarely the issues of health and healing that concern every one of us. He examines the most common causes of ill health and the reasons we fail to receive God's healing grace. Here we see how our Creator has lovingly provided all we need for wholeness of living, if only we set ourselves to live in accordance with his will.

Above all, this book shows that even when healing eludes us and our condition is not remedied quickly, we can still rest secure in the knowledge that our heavenly Father is committed to our good—in spirit, mind, emotions, and body.

Also by Selwyn Hughes in Kingsway paperback:
A friend in Need; How to Live the Christian Life; The Christian Counsellor's Pocket Guide; Everyday Reflections; A New Heart; Marriage as God Intended.

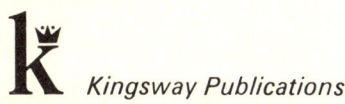

Kingsway Publications

The Healthy Alternative
Which way to wholeness?

by John Houghton

'Crowded city streets full of lonely people . . . hospitals and surgeries jam-packed . . . stress, violence and anxiety like jagged rocks cutting into the souls of millions . . .'

'Gentlemen, is there any cure for this malicious malady? Or shall society merely continue to put its trust in tranquillizers and television to ease this self-inflicted torment? What is to be done . . . ?'

   'That is what I have come to observe,' said the Pilgrim Watcher.

In a unique blend of fictional narrative and stimulating discussion, John Houghton brings together several imaginary characters who offer solutions to the ills of our materialistic Western society.

At the forefront of the story are Mr Aquarius and Mr Christian, both of whom reject the idea that man is just a complex machine. Each champions an alternative way of living, but it soon becomes apparent that they are irreconcilably different from each other. Mr Aquarius seeks to harmonize man and nature through various techniques and diets, while Mr Christian insists that the key to personal wholeness is a life centred on Jesus Christ and worked out in a Spirit-filled community.

As the narrative moves to a breathtaking climax, we are left with a prophetic challenge to seek answers from the source of true wholeness. Either way, we must decide.

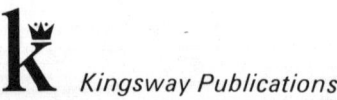

Kingsway Publications

Free to be Slim
A Christian Approach to Losing Weight

by Marie Chapian & Neva Coyle

You mustn't eat that...
   You can't eat that more than once a week.
      You must try harder...feel better
                     ...look younger.

Many books promise weight loss through rules, diets and techniques. This book adopts a radically new approach. Written for Christians who wish to change their eating habits, it goes to the root of the problem and deals with our motivation and lifestyle. Here we see that to lose weight must be seen as part of a whole process of offering our bodies to God. Then we can know victory in our lives as a reality and not just a hope.

Marie Chapian, working closely with Neva Coyle, has prepared this book from Neva's own weight-loss course. Neva herself has lost eight stone, and so the principles shared here are both realistic and encouraging.

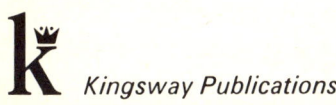

Kingsway Publications